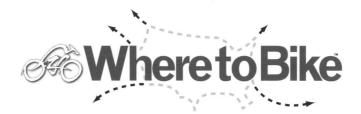

Where to Bike

Portland

- North/Northeast
- Downtown & Theme Rides
- West
- South
- East
- Kids' Rides

By Anne Lee

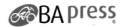
BA press

Where to Bike LLC

Email: mail@wheretobikeguides.com
Tel: +61 2 4274 4884 - Fax: +61 2 4274 0988
www.wheretobikeguides.com

First published in the USA in 2012 by Where to Bike LLC.

Design and Layout - Justine Powell
Advertising - Phil Latz
Photography - Matt Wittmer & Anne Lee
Mapping - Justine Powell, Bicycling Australia
Printed in China by RR Donnelley

Cover: Photo by Matt Wittmer

Library of Congress Control Number: 2012938395
Author: Anne Lee
Title: Where to Bike Portland
ISBN: 978-0-9871686-6-5
         978-0-9871686-9-6

The Cycling Kangaroo logo is a trademark of Lake Wangary Publishing Company Pty Ltd.

Where to Bike is a proud sponsor of World Bicycle Relief.

Where to Bike is a proud member of the Bikes Belong Coalition, organizers of the People for Bikes campaign; and the League of American Bicyclists.

peopleforbikes.org

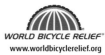

WORLD BICYCLE RELIEF®
www.worldbicyclerelief.org

League of
American
Bicyclists

www.bikeleague.org

Also in this series:
Where to Ride Melbourne
Where to Ride Adelaide
Where to Ride Perth
Where to Ride Sydney
Where to Ride Canberra
Where to Ride South East Queensland
Where to Ride Tasmania
Where to Ride Western & Northern Victoria
Where to Ride Eastern Victoria
Where to Ride Sydney MTB
Where to Ride London
Where to Bike Chicago
Where to Bike Washington, D.C.
Where to Bike Philadelphia
Where to Bike Los Angeles
Where to Bike New York City
Where to Bike Orange County
Where to Bike Los Angeles Mountain Biking

Coming soon:
Where to Ride Auckland
Where to Ride Melbourne Mountain Biking
Where to Bike Orange County Mountain Biking

Available on the
App Store

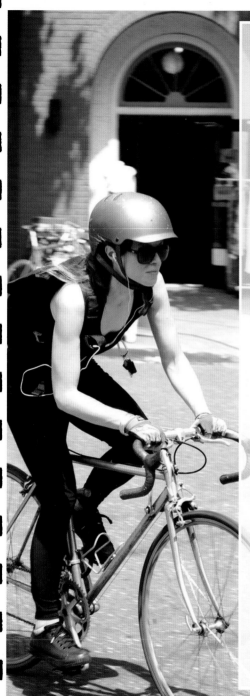

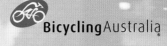
BicyclingAustralia

About us...

Cycling has many health and environmental benefits, but in addition to these it's a fun leisure time activity for all ages. Bike touring is also a great way to get up close and personal with a new destination. Where to Bike guides provide locals and tourists alike with advice on the best ride options for fun, exploration and relaxation on two wheels.

Most of our team are active cyclists; we love to ride and hope that we can inspire and motivate readers to join us on two wheels. We're committed to our vision of enhancing all aspects of cycling through these Where to Bike guides and our other publications.

Available in printed hard copy through bike shops and book stores, Where to Bike publications are also offered in digital format online. Check the iTunes store for an eBook version if you prefer a soft copy, or download the IOS App and we'll guide you along the route of each ride as you go!

Look out for other Where to Bike titles and the 'cycling kangaroo' logo in news stands and bookstores; it's your key to quality cycling publications.

We have made every effort to ensure the accuracy of the content of this book, but please feel free to contact us at feedback@wheretobikeguides.com to report any changes to routes or inconsistencies you may find.

For more information about *Where to Bike Portland* and other books in this series, visit **www.wheretobikeguides.com.**

Image Matt Wittmer

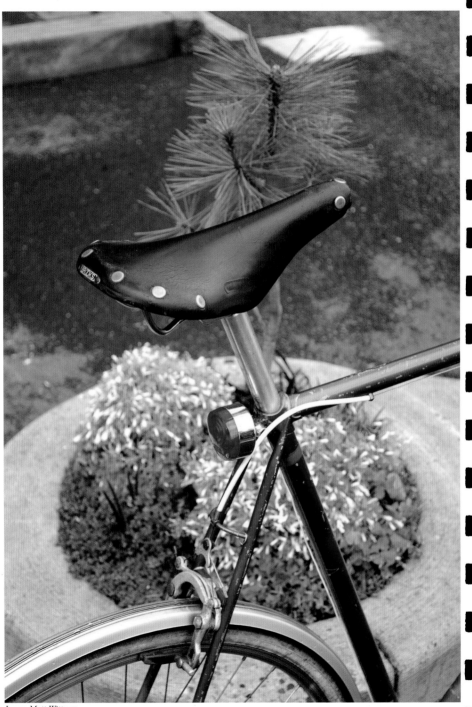

Image Matt Wittmer

Foreword by Mia Birk
President of Alta Planning & Design and Principal of Alta Bicycle Share, Inc.

Set off in the early morning dew on the Lincoln Street Bikeway and you will be in good company. Follow fellow cyclists' blinking red lights to downtown. Cross on one of our renovated bridges, marvel at the floating path on the Willamette River, then park your bike in one of thousands of covered, secure racks. Walk into a meeting holding your helmet and not one person will snort in amusement or derision. They've probably biked in themselves, if not today, another day. If not yet, soon. Take a deep breath and let your pulse rest, but know that you've started the day healthily, economically, safely.

It would be easy to think that the Portland, OR, we see today has always been the nation's number one bicycling city. Easy, but wrong. It didn't just happen. We made it happen. And it wasn't easy, as I recount in my book: *Joyride: Pedaling Toward a Healthier Planet*. Today, Portland's 325-miles of bikeways make bicycling a low-stress, low-cost, delightful option for many trips.

With this book, you'll discover the best, family-friendly routes. I adore riding on our lovely bicycle boulevards (a.k.a. neighborhood greenways,) such as SE Harrison/Lincoln up to Mount Tabor, NE Going Street, and NE Tillamook. Our off-street paths – Springwater Corridor, Peninsula Crossing Trail, Eastbank Esplanade, Willamette Greenway – are all wonderful. Make sure to head east on Marine Drive, the shimmering water of the Columbia to your left, a luminous Mount Hood straight ahead. Even our outlying and hillier parts of town have their opportunities and charms, all revealed in this book.

Summer in Portland is the perfect time to ride, but I've learned to appreciate our schizophrenic spring days, when I might get pelted by hail and then warmed by a double rainbow. Spring in Portland is stunning in its beauty, week after week offering new tantalizing eye candy: swirls of cherry blossoms, breathtaking lines of white ornamental pear trees, pink Magnolia explosion, and a dazzling array of yellow, green, pink, white, and purple Camellias, Dogwoods, and Rhododendrons. You just don't get the same level of flowery intoxication sitting in a car. In fall, we get the autumn colors, and in winter, well ... you just never know.

As you explore Portland by bike, please model good behavior. Always wait for red lights, yield to pedestrians, and slow and prepare to stop at stop signs. As you'll find, many motorists will wave at you to proceed first, even though they have the right-of-way. Accept these moments of grace for what they are: a gift of understanding. Probably they themselves ride from time to time. Your responsibility: accept the gift, and smile and wave in gratitude. And since this will happen often, you'll find yourself smiling and waving, waving and smiling, happy, happy, happy as you pedal along, until you arrive at your destination feeling pleasantly hungry, energetic, filled with joy.

Enjoy the ride!

> *"Today, Portland's 325-miles of bikeways make bicycling a low-stress, low-cost, delightful option for many trips".*

Mia Birk

President, Alta Planning & Design
Principal, Alta Bicycle Share, Inc.

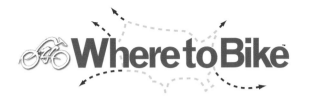

Portland

Contents

About Us 3
Foreword..5
Author's Note 10
About the Author.. 11
Introduction 12
How to Use This Book 14
Terrain Guide 16
Before You Go/What to Take 17
Ride Overview.. 18-21
World Bicycle Relief... 22
On the Road 24
You, Your Bike and Transport in Portland 26
Public Transport Maps 28-31
About the Community Cycling Center 32
Notes.. 278
Bike Shops & Rentals in and around Portland 282

North/Northeast

Introduction 40
Ride 1 - Clark County Tour... 44
Ride 2 - Fort Vancouver to Lacamas Lake 48
Ride 3 - Fort Vancouver to Vancouver Lake 52
Ride 4 - Vancouver Maritime Trail....................................... 56
Ride 5 - Downtown Vancouver to the Airport 60
Ride 6 - Two Bridges Two States Loop 64
Ride 7 - Columbia Tech Center 68
Ride 8 - Sauvie Island... 72
Ride 9 - Smith and Bybee Lakes to Kelley Point Park...... 76
Ride 10 - St. Johns Loop.. 80
Ride 11 - Walls of Pride Art Loop 84
Ride 12 - Fernhill Park.. 88
Ride 13 - Ground Water Well Tour 92
Ride 14 - Cully Neighborhood Figure Eight 96

Downtown & Theme Rides

Introduction 104
Ride 15 - Museums by Bike.. 108
Ride 16 - Willamette Bridges Tour 112
Ride 17 - Heritage Tree Tour.. 116
Ride 18 - Tri-Park Trip 120
Ride 19 - Architectural Ride 124
Ride 20 - The Doughnut Roll 128
Ride 21 - Water Water Everywhere Fountain Ride.. 132
Ride 22 - Bike-Friendly Brewery Tour... 136
Ride 23 - Tour of the Food Carts 140
Ride 24 - The Simpsons Ride.. 144
Ride 25 - Garden Tour 148
Ride 26 - Public Art Ride 152
Ride 27 - Crazy Parks Ride 156
Ride 28 - PSU to Ladd's Addition... 160
Ride 29 - Downtown Portland to the Airport.. 164

West

Introduction 168
Ride 30 - Vista Bridge to Council Crest Park.. 172
Ride 31 - Pittock Mansion to Council Crest via Washington Park 176
Ride 32 - Cedar Hills to Sylvan Hills 180
Ride 33 - Hillsboro to Vernonia 184
Ride 34 - Hillsboro Stroll 188
Ride 35 - Jackson Bottom Loop 192
Ride 36 - Hillsboro Farmlands 196

South

Introduction 200
Ride 37 - Wine Country via Chehalem Mountain.. 204
Ride 38 - Champoeg State Park 208
Ride 39 - Terwilliger Boulevard to Lake Oswego via Tryon State Park 212
Ride 40 - Clackamas River Ride.. 216

East

Introduction 222
Ride 41 - Rocky Mount Ride... 226
Ride 42 - East Portland Loop Ride.. 230
Ride 43 - Knead the Dough 234
Ride 44 - Marine Drive to Troutdale Loop 238
Ride 45 - I-205 Bike Path to Clackamas Town Center 242
Ride 46 - Columbia River Gorge to Multnomah Falls....................................... 246

Kids' Rides

Introduction 250

North/Northeast
Ride K1 - Burnt Bridge Creek Trail.. 252
Ride K2 - Esther Short Park.. 253
Ride K3 - Washington State University Park................................. 254
Ride K4 - Salmon Creek Trail... 255
Ride K5 - Kelley Point Park.. 256
Ride K6 - Blue Lake Regional Park.. 257
Ride K7 - Cathedral City Park.. 258
Ride K8 - Columbia Park.. 259
Ride K9 - Wellington Park.. 260
Ride K10 - Peninsula Park.. 261
Ride K11 - Pier Park... 262
Ride K12 - Overlook Park... 263
Ride K13 - Wallace City Park... 264
Ride K14 - McKenna Park.. 265
Ride K15 - Dawson City Park.. 266
Ride K16 - Alberta Park... 267
Ride K17 - Tanner Springs Park.. 268
Ride K18 - Irving Park.. 269

Southeast
Ride K19 - Laurelhurst Park.. 270
Ride K20 - OMSI to Sellwood Park.. 271
Ride K21 - East Esplanade to OMSI... 272
Ride K22 - Grant Park.. 273

West
Ride K23 - Greenway Park at Fanno Creek 274
Ride K24 - Tualatin Hills Nature Park 275
Ride K25 - Shute Park.. 276
Ride K26 - Rood Bridge Park 277

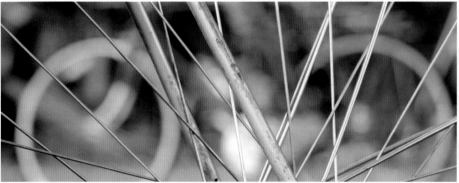

Image Matt Wittmer

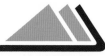
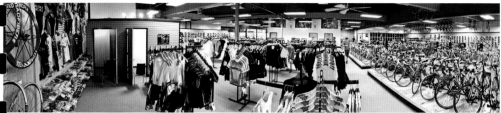
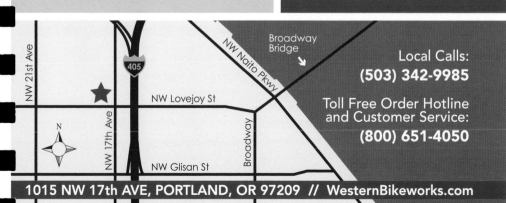

Author's Note

Though locals may enjoy bicycling around their city, visitors will find this book a terrific way to discover Portland – the sights, the art, the beer, the surrounding countryside, and the quirkiness of this wonderful city.

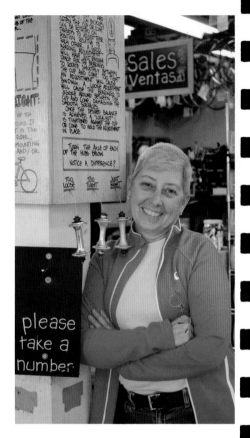

Portland and its surrounds offer what seem to be a limitless number of wonderful bike rides and the most daunting aspect of writing this book was culling the choices down to a manageable number. Through the 5,000 miles of riding and writing this book, I have come to know more than just how to navigate the city. Bicycling allows one to hear the heartbeat of the city – a beautiful place with incredibly passionate and creative people – who have embraced bicycling as a way of life. Come explore this place rolling along at 12 miles per hour and discover Portland for the first time.

Many bicyclists in Portland keep to the comfort of their familiar neighborhood, their bike train to school, or their commute to work. I invite you to consider this book a guide for locals to explore beyond your neighborhood or that one summer excursion to the coast you may look forward to all winter. Take a Sunday afternoon with family and friends and visit volcanoes and summits, or consider an arts and entertainment ride. This book will bring you to gardens bursting with color, to breweries with as many as 50 taps, to food carts that make the mouth water, and more. Share your adventures with others and plan new ones of your own.

Instead of spending time poring over maps to find the perfect route, I found it more important to let the ride evolve along the way. Infrastructure changes are common in Portland, especially in the downtown area and on the east side of the Willamette River where bicycles are concentrated. Even the best plan must allow for adjustments and I encourage you to consider the road construction you will undoubtedly encounter as a precursor to improved bicycle infrastructure.

While exploring Oregon is intriguing, I have confined myself to Portland and its surrounding areas in order to highlight the incredible scenery and surprising beauty of this small corner of the northwest. It sometimes pained me to have to choose one particular route over another and to cull the hundreds of photos down to the few that appear in these pages. Now you can use these routes and photos to create your own scrapbook of adventures and discoveries, and marvel at the wonderful place that is Portland.

Ride safe!

Anne F Lee

Anne Lee
Author & Photographer

About the Author

Anne Lee's first bicycle was a shiny blue beauty with a white seat and stripes along the fenders. It seemed to dwarf the tree it stood beside on Christmas morning. In the northeast winter takes its time saying goodbye, but that first warm spring day when the sidewalk was finally clear of snow, a small child found freedom and adventure on her new bike. That bicycle took Lee on many excursions growing up. The joy she found as a child compelled Lee to graduate from recreational cyclist to a full-fledged bicycle commuter when she moved to the west coast.

Lee grew up in Boston, earned her undergraduate degree from Emmanuel College, and her Master's degree from the University of Southern Maine. After a career in banking, Lee and three other colleagues became publishers of a weekly help-wanted newspaper with circulation in Maine and New Hampshire. Even the adventures of building a company from the ground up did not hold her interest beyond five years. Lee joined the YWCA and turned her attention toward nonprofit management.

After spending a year in South Carolina attending to family matters, Lee turned west and chose Portland, Oregon as her home because of the city's commitment to urban planning, sustainability, and bicycling. She joined the Community Cycling Center where she applies her business sense to the mission of broadening access to bicycles and hangs her helmet between bicycle adventures.

Gratitude

No measure of thanks could possibly be enough to express my gratitude for those people who assisted in developing and riding the thousands of miles that have become this book. I feel enormously thankful for Joseph Greulich, the trusted companion on many of the rides you'll find here. Thanks, too, to Robert Wenz, a cycling newbie whose enthusiasm is contagious. I could not have maintained my dedication to this work without the support and encouragement of the Community Cycling Center. The final edition you hold in your hands would not be possible without the hours of dedicated proofreading and editing of the wonderful crew at Bicycling Australia, Joanne and Justine. Karen Mathieson of Serendipity Communications and Roy Wilkinson were welcome coaches for final edits. But my most heartfelt thanks go to the local champions and advocates who have passionately nurtured the bicycle culture of Portland and who make this the Platinum City it is.

Photography

Many thanks to **Matt Wittmer**, author and photographer of the inspiring *Where to Bike Washington, D.C.*, who assisted in creation of this book by capturing additional images to compliment those taken by Anne Lee.

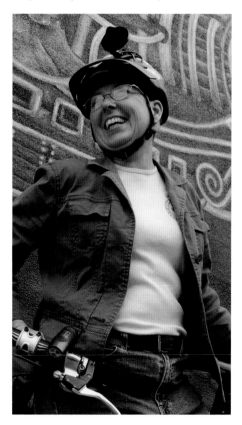

Introduction

Between these pages you will find 46 adult and 26 kids' rides centered in the greater Portland area within a radius of about 35 miles. The adult rides begin and end at public transportation points and many have access to bus routes and/or MAX trains within a reasonable distance. The kids' rides are short and centered in parks and bicycle-dedicated pathways. Many rides take you over the well-planned roads of bicycle infrastructure for which Portland has become famous. Others travel through rural areas where cyclists and automobiles share the road.

By traveling the rides outlined in the five sections of this book you will get to know the area in all its glory. From the steep West Hills to the wildlife refuge in Ridgefield; from historic Champoeg State Park to the diagonal streets of Ladd's Addition; from wine country made famous by vintners of world-class Pinot Noir to the elegant St. John's Bridge; from the mighty Columbia to the Willamette River that bisects Portland, this book helps you explore it all.

Fourteen rides north and northeast of Portland traverse two states and much of the beauty of rivers, neighborhoods, and rural Washington State. The next 15 centered in downtown Portland give a flavor of the unique gifts of the city by highlighting food, beer, and culture, not to mention the very practical cycling routes to the airport. Next, get your heart pumping by riding through the West Hills, find breathtaking views of mountain ranges and enchanting neighborhoods, then head further west to farm country. South of the city connect with the region's earliest history and sample the fruits of wine country. Turning east and riding through the Gorge by waterfalls and over spent volcanoes highlights the geologic formations that give this area its stunning beauty.

Adult rides are designed to take advantage of bicycle infrastructure around the area as well as points of interest along the way. Many of the adult rides are perfectly suitable for families with children who are confident cycling on the road. For those who are not quite road-ready, the last section of the book is designed for kids just beginning their bicycling journeys.

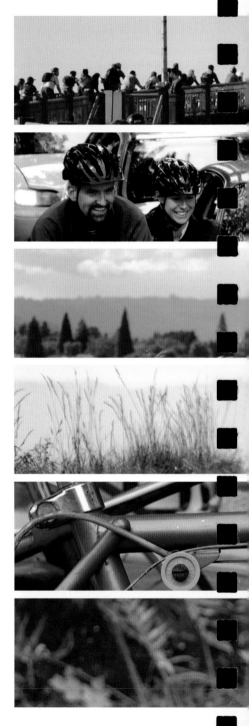

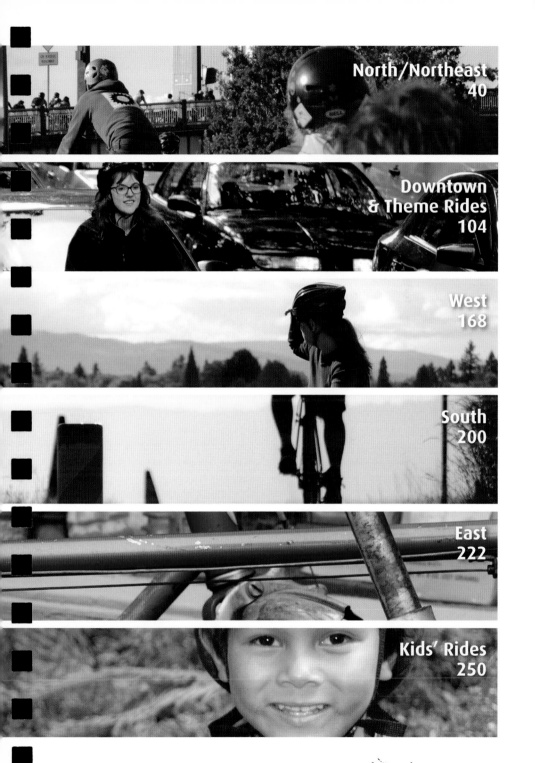

North/Northeast
40

Downtown & Theme Rides
104

West
168

South
200

East
222

Kids' Rides
250

How to Use this Book

In *Where to Bike Portland* you will find 72 ways for adults and kids to explore the region. The rides are divided into six sections: North/Northeast, Downtown & Theme Rides, West, South, East and Kids' Rides, the latter of which includes rides in each geographic area.

Most of the rides are on bike paths, bike lanes, and paved streets that run over smooth surfaces. Many rides use urban and neighborhood streets, bike boulevards, or have painted bike sharrows (share-the-road arrows) designating them as "bike friendly" routes. This system is designed to make your initial selection quick and easy based on the terrain you are likely to encounter along the way.

Ride Scale

To help you better understand how difficult each ride might be, this book uses a riding scale developed by the publisher, Bicycling Australia, for all its bicycle guidebooks. Each ride is assigned points based on the total distance, the elevation gain, and the predominant road surface. The points are added up to determine the overall rating. You can find the Where to Bike rating

on the introductory page of each ride; just look for the Bicycling Australia kangaroo symbols:

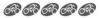

The Where to Bike rating is only a guide. If you are new to cycling or just getting into shape, start with level one and two rides. As your cycling skills improve, you will be able to challenge yourself with the more advanced rides. You will find that most of the level one and two rides are suitable for doing as a family.

While the maps have been produced with accurate GPS-collected data, they do not always show sufficient detail to allow you to navigate relying exclusively on them. That is where the ride logs before each map come in. Refer to the logs as you bike since they provide the information and detail you need to get from start to finish.

Make sure you also use the specially designed inside front cover to keep you on the right page. This fold-out flap also includes the key to the maps and introductory pages. There are a few pages at the back of the book to add your own notes about the rides or places you would like to revisit.

We hope all of these design features will ensure that you enjoy rides that are safe and carefree, informative and entertaining.

	1 pt	2 pts	3 pts	4 pts	5 pts
Distance – Road (miles)	<12	12-19	19-25	25-37	>37
Distance – MTB (miles)	<6	6-9	9-16	16-25	>25
Climbing (feet)	<500	500 - 1,000	1,000 - 1,500	1,500 - 2,000	>2,000
Surface	Paved smooth	Paved rough	Unpaved smooth	Unpaved moderate	Unpaved rough

Accumulated Points	Riding Level/Grade	Suggested Suitability
3	1	Beginner
4-5	2	
6-7	3	Moderately fit
8-9	4	
10+	5	Experienced cyclist

Ride Classifications

Ride Classifications are used to represent the distinct character of the ride itself and are usually a reflection of the environment or landscape the cyclist will enjoy as they travel the route.

In *Where to Bike Portland*, there are eight classifications to look for on the ride At a Glance page:

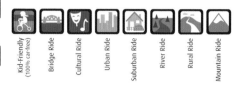

Kid-Friendly (100% car-free) | Bridge Ride | Cultural Ride | Urban Ride | Suburban Ride | River Ride | Rural Ride | Mountain Ride

Ride Links

If you're partial to adding to your ride, or simply interested in other routes nearby, information on ride links can be found on both the ride At a Glance page, and on the maps.

At a Glance: Ride numbers included in the 'Links to' panel on the At a Glance page are considered direct links—rides that intersect with, or can be accessed with ease from the current route.

Maps: Each map includes easy to identify ride link icons. The maps show all links, both direct and non-direct—direct links appear along the route of the current ride at the location of junction, while indirect routes appear at a distance at their start location. Refer to the linked ride pages to hop on board another route to extend your ride or to visit a previously undiscovered Portland neighborhood.

Bike Shops and Rentals

Bike shops and bike rental outlets are marked upon each map with icons as above. Each icon carries a number which correlates to a comprehensive store listing on page 282. Here you'll find the name, number and web details of the stores that are an easy pedal from all of the rides. No spares? No worries.

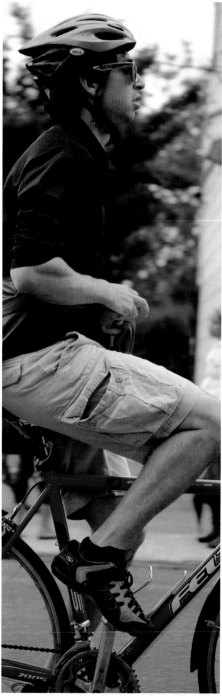

Image Matt Wittmer

Terrain Guide

To help you understand what to expect on the route, terrain types are described on both the At a Glance page, and directly on the maps with easy to follow colored ride lines, as follows:

On-Road:

A *red ride line* depicts sections of the ride that are on-road. The cyclist shares the road with vehicular traffic, and is expected to abide by road rules and laws. These routes are either Class III Bike Routes, or are considered comparably safe for recommendation by the author.

Neighborhood Greenway:

A *purple ride line* depicts sections of the ride that are on Neighborhood Greenways. Here the cyclist travels residential streets with low volumes of auto traffic and low speeds where bicycle and pedestrians are given priority. They are indicated by pavement markings, or sharrows (share-the-road arrows), and directional signs to guide cyclists. They usually contain additional traffic-calming features such as speed bumps and extended curbs. These routes are only indicated if such infrastructure is in place.

On-Road Bike Lane:

A *green ride line* depicts sections of the ride where exclusive on-road bike lanes are provided. Here the cyclist is clearly separated from vehicular traffic by a traffic lane marked on an existing roadway that is restricted to cycle traffic. These routes are Class II Bike Routes, and are only indicated if such infrastructure is in place.

Protected On-Road Bike Lane:

A *blue ride line* depicts sections of the ride where exclusive, protected on-road bike lanes are provided. Here the cyclist is clearly separated from vehicular traffic by a physical barrier that is restricted to use by cycle traffic. Such barriers can consist of parked cars or painted curbs. These routes are also considered Class I Bike Routes, and are only indicated if such infrastructure is in place.

Designated Bike Path:

A *yellow ride line* depicts sections of the ride that are on smooth bike paths where the cyclist is completely separated from roads. The path can either be a sidepath (designated for use by cyclists) or a shared-use footway (for use by both cyclists and pedestrians). These routes are either Class I Bike Routes, or are considered comparably safe for recommendation by the author.

Before You Go

The benefits of cycling as part of a healthy lifestyle and recreational pastime are obvious, but if you are a novice cyclist or resuming cycling after a long hiatus, consult your doctor with any health concerns before you venture out.

It is also wise to ensure that your bicycle and equipment are in good working order before heading out. Here are the main things to do:

- Inflate tires to the suggested air pressure.
- Inspect tires for damage or anything that might be embedded in the tread.
- Check the brake pads and cables.
- Make certain that the gear cables are tight and that every gear works.
- Ensure that the chain is clean and lubricated.
- Install bike lights on front and rear; make sure the batteries are fresh.

Of course, the best time to take care of all this is between outings. If you are unsure about any of these points, visit a bike shop for advice or service. There are many in Portland. Once you are ready to leave, let somebody know where you are planning to ride and how long you are likely to be away.

What to Take

On most rides in this book you are never far from civilization. Nevertheless, make sure that you've got everything you need before leaving.

Essentials

- Bicycle helmet with correctly adjusted straps.
- Spare inner tube, tire levers, and perhaps, a puncture repair kit.
- Bicycle pump or gas canister.
- Multi-use tool and any other tools specific to your bike.

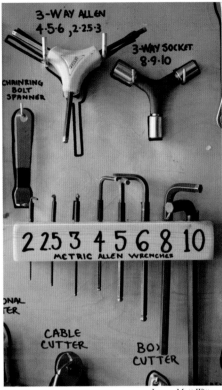

Image Matt Wittmer

- Sunscreen.
- Plenty of water; one quart per hour is recommended.
- Snacks to keep your blood sugar level up.
- Cell phone and/or phone card.
- Identification.
- Small first aid kit.
- Money.
- Information about any medical condition.
- Bicycle lock.
- Lights.

Optional

- Compact poncho or rain jacket (always a good idea in Portland during winter and spring).
- Camera.
- Binoculars.
- Bell installed on handlebars.
- Fenders will keep you dry.

Ride Overview

North/Northeast

Page	Ride	Ride Name	Start Location
44	1	Clark County Tour	Downtown Vancouver
48	2	Fort Vancouver to Lacamas Lake	Expo MAX Station, Portland
52	3	Fort Vancouver to Vancouver Lake	Downtown Vancouver
56	4	Vancouver Maritime Trail	Downtown Vancouver
60	5	Downtown Vancouver to the Airport	Downtown Vancouver
64	6	Two Bridges Two States Loop	Expo MAX Station, Portland
68	7	Columbia Tech Center	Columbia Valley Elementary School, Vancouver
72	8	Sauvie Island	N Gillihan Road, Sauvie Island
76	9	Smith and Bybee Lakes to Kelley Point Park	Rose Quarter MAX Station, Portland
80	10	St. Johns Loop	NE Failing St. and MLK Blvd., Portland
84	11	Walls of Pride Art Loop	NE Seventh Ave. MAX Station, Portland
88	12	Fernhill Park	NE Going St. and MLK Blvd., Portland
92	13	Ground Water Well Tour	Cascade MAX Station, Portland
96	14	Cully Neighborhood Figure Eight	Rigler Elementary School, Portland

Downtown & Theme Rides

Page	Ride	Ride Name	Start Location
108	15	Museums by Bike	SW Park Street and SW Jefferson Street, Portland
112	16	Willamette Bridges Tour	Union Station, Portland
116	17	Heritage Tree Tour	Wellington Park, Portland
120	18	Tri-Park Trip	Laurelhurst Park, Portland
124	19	Architectural Ride	Rose Quarter MAX Station, Portland
128	20	The Doughnut Roll	Union Station, Portland
132	21	Water Water Everywhere Fountain Ride	SW Morrison Street and SW 3rd Avenue, Portland
136	22	Bike-Friendly Brewery Tour	SW 18th Avenue and SW Salmon Street, Portland
140	23	Tour of the Food Carts	SW Morrison Street and SW 3rd Avenue, Portland
144	24	The Simpsons Ride	Washington Park MAX Station, Portland
148	25	Garden Tour	Rose Quarter MAX Station, Portland
152	26	Public Art Ride	Union Station, Portland
156	27	Crazy Parks Ride	Washington Park MAX Station, Portland
160	28	PSU to Ladd's Addition	SW Harrison Street and SW 6th Avenue, Portland
164	29	Downtown Portland to the Airport	Union Station, Portland

Terrain		Kid-Friendly	Distance (miles)	Elev. Gain (feet)	WTB Rating
On Road / On Road Lane		no	40.4	3295	
On Road / On Road Lane / Path		no	40.4	1440	
On Road / On Road Lane / Path		partial	18.8	306	
On Road / On Road Lane / Path		partial	11.6	425	
On Road Lane / Path		partial	11.0	240	
On Road / On Road Lane / Path		partial	20.7	720	
On Road / On Road Lane / Path		partial	2.95	20	
On Road		no	38.2	365	
On Road / On Road Lane / Path		partial	27.7	735	
On Road / Greenway / On Road Lane / Path		no	15.0	455	
On Road / Greenway / On Road Lane		no	10.7	540	
On Road / Greenway		no	9.2	340	
On Road / On Road Lane / Path		no	15.4	280	
On Road / On Road Lane		no	6.9	385	

Terrain		Kid-Friendly	Distance (miles)	Elev. Gain (feet)	WTB Rating
On Road / Greenway / On Road Lane		no	10.6	622	
On Road / Greenway / On Road Lane / Path		partial	26.6	1078	
On Road / Greenway / On Road Lane		no	9.2	262	
On Road / Greenway		no	6.2	260	
On Road / Greenway / On Road Lane		no	9.1	535	
On Road / Greenway / On Road Lane / Path		partial	17.7	850	
On Road / On Road Lane / Path		partial	3.92	320	
On Road / Greenway / On Road Lane / Protected Ln		no	11.2	505	
On Road / Greenway / On Road Lane / Path		no	13.5	635	
On Road / On Road Lane / Path		no	34.9	2800	
On Road / Greenway / On Road Lane / Path		partial	16.0	890	
On Road / Greenway / On Road Lane / Path		no	7.1	420	
On Road / Greenway / On Road Lane / Path		no	13.0	1614	
On Road / Greenway / On Road Lane / Path		no	11.2	665	
On Road / Greenway / On Road Lane / Path		no	10.3	490	

Ride Overview continued

West

Page	Ride	Ride Name	Start Location
172	30	Vista Bridge to Council Crest Park	Goose Hollow MAX Station, Portland
176	31	Pittock Mansion to Council Crest Park via Washington Park	SW 61st Drive, Portland
180	32	Cedar Hills to Sylvan Hills	Beaverton Transit Center MAX Station, Beaverton
184	33	Hillsboro to Vernonia	Hillsboro Government Center MAX Station, Hillsboro
188	34	Hillsboro Stroll	Hillsboro Government Center MAX Station, Hillsboro
192	35	Jackson Bottom Loop	Hillsboro Government Center MAX Station, Hillsboro
196	36	Hillsboro Farmlands	Orenco MAX Station, Hillsboro

South

Page	Ride	Ride Name	Start Location
204	37	Wine Country via Chehalem Mountain	Hillsboro Government Center MAX Station, Hillsboro
208	38	Champoeg State Park	Beaverton Transit Center MAX Station, Beaverton
212	39	Terwilliger Blvd to Lake Oswego via Tryon State Park	SW Columbia Street and SW Broadway, Portland
216	40	Clackamas River Ride	End of the Trail Interpretive Center, Oregon City

East

Page	Ride	Ride Name	Start Location
226	41	Rocky Mount Ride	Rose Quarter MAX Station, Portland
230	42	East Portland Loop Ride	Rose Quarter MAX Station, Portland
234	43	Knead the Dough	Rose Quarter MAX Station, Portland
238	44	Marine Drive to Troutdale Loop	Expo MAX Station, Portland
242	45	I-205 Bike Path to Clackamas Town Center	NE Going St. and MLK Blvd., Portland
246	46	Columbia River Gorge to Multnomah Falls	Glenn Otto Community Park, Troutdale

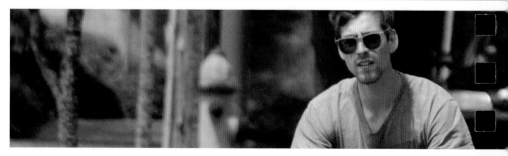

Terrain				Kid-Friendly	Distance (miles)	Elev. Gain (feet)	WTB Rating
On Road / On Road Lane				no	9.7	1538	
On Road / On Road Lane / Path				no	14.0	2369	
On Road / On Road Lane / Path				partial	6.7	430	
On Road / Path				partial	70.64	5390	
On Road / On Road Lane / Path				no	41.6	1790	
On Road / On Road Lane				no	21.6	1423	
On Road / On Road Lane				no	38.4	1750	

Terrain				Kid-Friendly	Distance (miles)	Elev. Gain (feet)	WTB Rating
On Road / On Road Lane				no	52.0	3950	
On Road / On Road Lane / Path				partial	52.9	2416	
On Road / On Road Lane / Path				partial	25.0	2760	
On Road				no	25.0	1700	

Terrain				Kid-Friendly	Distance (miles)	Elev. Gain (feet)	WTB Rating
On Road / Greenway / On Road Lane / Path				partial	20.6	1497	
On Road / Greenway / On Road Lane / Path				partial	32.7	1170	
On Road / Greenway / On Road Lane / Path				partial	19.8	960	
On Road / On Road Lane / Path				partial	36.4	835	
On Road / Greenway / On Road Lane / Path				partial	35.3	1830	
On Road / On Road Lane				no	35.9	2714	

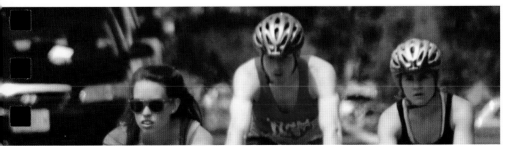

Image Matt Wittmer

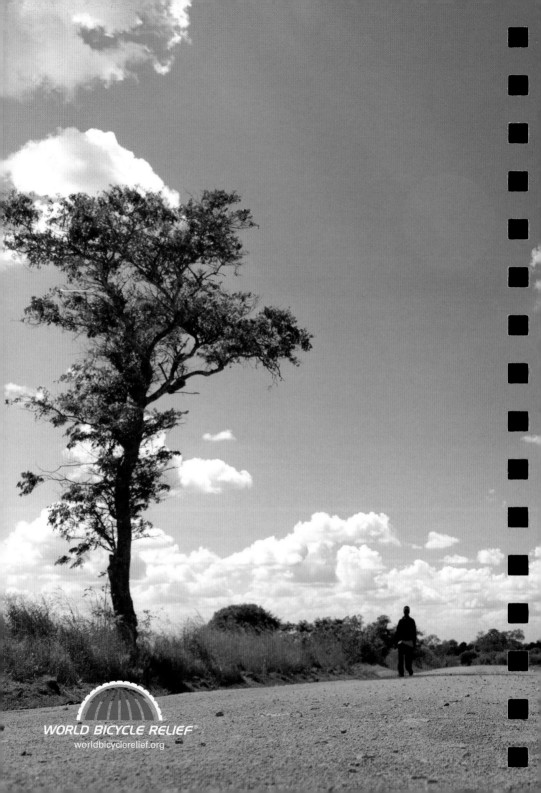

WORLD BICYCLE RELIEF®
worldbicyclerelief.org

teacher. doctor. engineer…

This bicycle is more than transportation;
it's a new beginning.
worldbicyclerelief.org/pages/newbeginning

On the Road

It is not pleasant to think about the dangers of cycling. Even though Portland is a Platinum City and bicycles are everywhere, accidents and serious injuries are still a concern when riding a bicycle in the greater Portland area. A study by the Oregon Health and Science University (OHSU) in 2010 indicated that one in five Portland bicycle commuters will be involved in a bicycle accident resulting in personal injury. The good news is that there is a lot you can do to avoid becoming a statistic.

The single most important thing is to *always wear a helmet* – even on bike trails where automobile traffic may be the last thing on your mind. Oregon law requires helmets for riders under the age of 16. Also wear brightly colored clothing and have a headlight attached to your helmet. Install lights on your bike – a white light on the handlebars and a red blinking light on the rear. Reflectors are not usually enough, and do not meet the legal requirements. If you find yourself out beyond dusk or in limited visibility conditions, lights are required.

Remember that you are in traffic. Bike in a predictable fashion. Don't weave in and out of parked cars. Ride in the direction of traffic, staying in your lane, signaling your intention to turn, and stopping at red lights and stop signs. "Share the Road" is not just a catchy slogan: it is the law in Oregon. At some intersections there are bicycle traffic signals in addition to automobile traffic signals to direct all vehicles safely. Though bicycles have the right-of-way over automobiles, defensive cycling is always a safer way to negotiate streets. In Oregon the law also requires bicyclists to give the right-of-way to pedestrians, even when they are not in a painted, designated crosswalk. The safest way to cycle is to follow the "eye-to-eye" rule. When you can look the automobile drivers and pedestrians in the eye, you are better able to indicate your intentions, as are they.

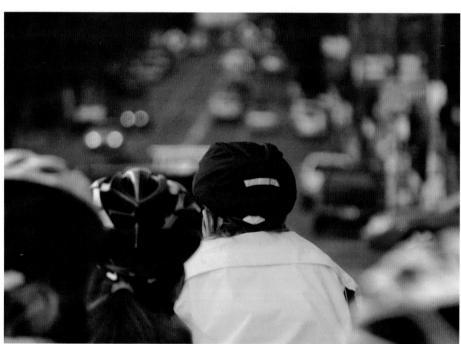

Image Matt Wittmer

Here are some finer points of bike safety:

- If you stop, move off the path.
- Do not go fast on crushed stone paths no matter how smooth they may be; that way you will avoid the possibility of hitting a soft spot and having a collision.
- Bicycle on the right, pass on the left. Whenever you pass someone, bicyclist or pedestrian, say "on your left" or ring your bell before passing.
- Ride single file when the path is crowded. Some bike lanes allow for two-abreast riding, but single file is safer and preferable.
- Yield to pedestrians and skaters.
- Yield to horses and call out a greeting as you approach a horse from behind so that it will hear you coming and not get spooked.
- Watch out for the "right hook" where a car turns right just ahead of you.
- Avoid getting "doored" (being hit by a car door that opens unexpectedly) by riding at least three feet away from parked and stopped cars when possible.
- When going straight through an intersection with a turning lane, position yourself to the closest lane going straight.
- When there is a green painted "bike box" in the street, it will provide the right of way at traffic signals to bicycles in the form of a space in front of automobiles.
- Use your bike bell! Automobiles have lots of blind spots. You can provide yourself a safer ride if you announce yourself with your bell.
- Get a rearview mirror for your handlebars or helmet.
- In Oregon, bicycles are vehicles and must obey vehicle laws. When in doubt, dismount your bike and use pedestrian crossing signals.
- Driving Under the Influence (DUI) laws apply when you are riding your bicycle.
- Bicycles are allowed to ride in the traffic lane when the lane is narrow or when you are traveling at the same speed as the traffic. When a bike lane is available, riders must use it except when necessary to safely turn, pass, or avoid a hazard.
- Cross railroad tracks at a right angle to the tracks.
- Traffic signals are triggered by electrically charged wires buried under the pavement. Look for cut lines in the pavement filled with tar. There is usually enough metal in the bike to trip the light.
- Never make a left turn from the right lane. Use designated turn lanes when possible. Use a "box style turn" when necessary. Ride through the intersection on the right side of the road. Make a 90 degree left turn and proceed as if you were approaching the intersection from the right.
- Use hand signals.
- Hold your arm straight out in the direction you intend to turn.
- Right turns can be signaled by holding your left arm up with bent elbow.
- Signal stopping by holding your left arm down with bent elbow.

You will actually enhance your safety by claiming your place on the road with confidence and even a bit of assertiveness. You have every right to be on the road, as long as you follow the rules.

At the same time, a little courtesy goes a long way. If motorists see you cycling in a responsible fashion, they will be more likely to respond in kind – and to develop a positive image of bicycling for the next time they encounter you or another cyclist. Whenever and wherever you cycle, you are an ambassador for all things bicycle.

For Oregon laws governing bicycles, consult the Oregon Department of Transportation Oregon Bicyclist Manual.

You, Your Bike and Transport in Portland

Greater Portland and surrounding counties are fortunate to have a vast, comprehensive public transportation system that accommodates bicycles. Get to know the system and you'll find that it will take you and your bike almost anywhere around the region comfortably, conveniently, and cheaply. In addition, public transportation provides a great backup in case it rains, you have gone too far, or you have mechanical problems that you cannot or would rather not fix on the road.

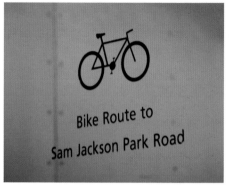

Image Matt Wittmer

Putting your bike on the bus is easy. Buses are equipped with a bike rack on the front that accommodates two bicycles. When the bike rack is full, which happens more and more, it is best to simply wait for the next bus. To put your bike on the bus, the rack must be lowered using the handle in the middle just on the inside of the rack. Squeeze the handle up and the rack will release. The bike racks are heavy, so it is best to have both hands available. Lift your bike into the groove. One bike will face the sidewalk (inside position closest to the bus), and one bike will face the street (outside position furthest away from the bus). Once your bike is positioned on the rack, lift the bar onto your front tire to hold the bike in place. Remove any bags or loose items from the bike as the bus driver will not stop if your gear goes flying. When you are ready to leave the bus, be sure to tell the bus driver that you need to get your bike. You cannot expect the driver to remember which riders have bikes mounted on the front of the bus, and it is safer to announce the fact that you will be stepping in front of the bus. If yours is the only bike being removed, lift the rack and push to lock it into place. If you and another cyclist are both taking the bus from the same station, it is polite to ask where the other cyclist is disembarking. The cyclist who is staying on the bus longer will mount his/her bike on the inside position for ease of the other cyclist removing his/her bicycle.

Putting your bike on the train, known as the MAX, is easier. Most trains are equipped with bike hooks at the front and rear of the train behind passenger seats. Just roll your bike onto the train and you will see the hooks designated for your bike. These hooks are often occupied by other bikes, and when this happens, you will simply stand with your bike among the passengers in the least intrusive manner possible. Passengers are usually accommodating of bicyclists and try to give a wide berth. You may also find it easier to exit if you announce to the other passengers that you are exiting with a bicycle. They will give you a clear exit path.

There is no extra charge for taking your bike. Public transportation in the greater Portland area is very accessible and easy to negotiate. Many of the rides in the book can be done using public transportation to the start point or along the way.

If you are spending time in Portland you may want to make note of the Time Tracker, an electronic system designed to help you find real-time arrival times of buses throughout the TriMet transit system. The number to call to access the system is 503-238-7433, or you can download a variety of free and commercial transit applications for your smart phone from the website. Alternatively, you can find all the information you need to travel by public transportation by visiting TriMet at **www.trimet.org**.

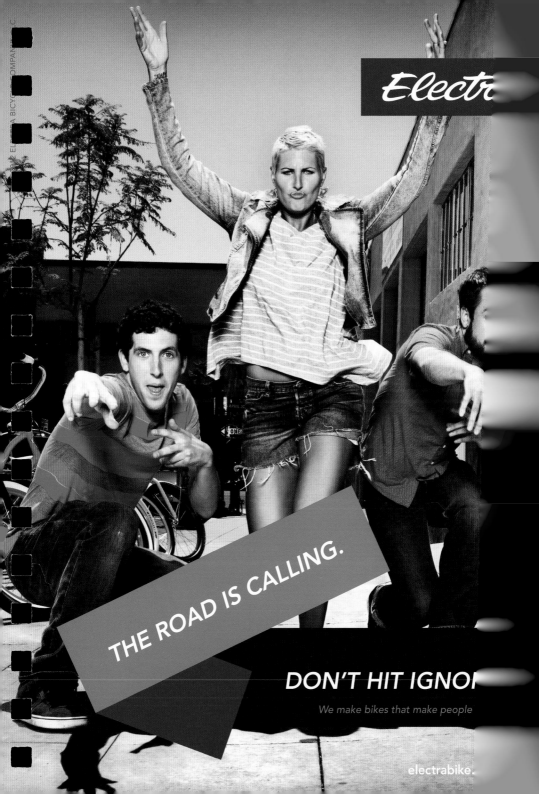

Portland City Center and Rail Zone

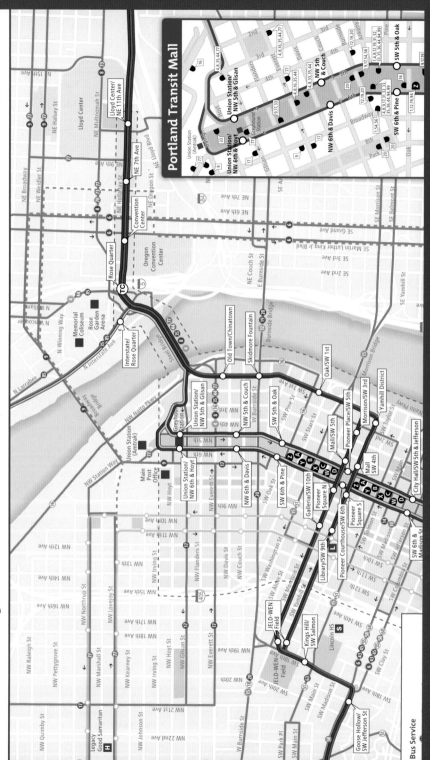

TRI❍MET

Portland Transit Mall

Bus Service

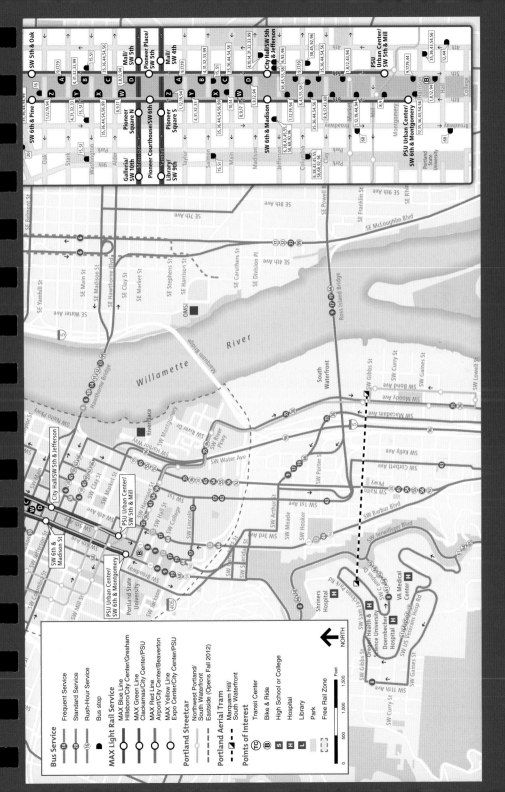

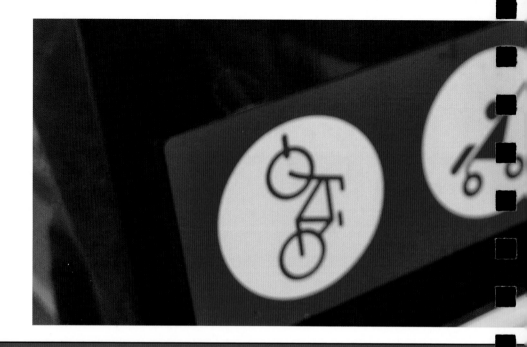

TRI🌀MET
Rail System

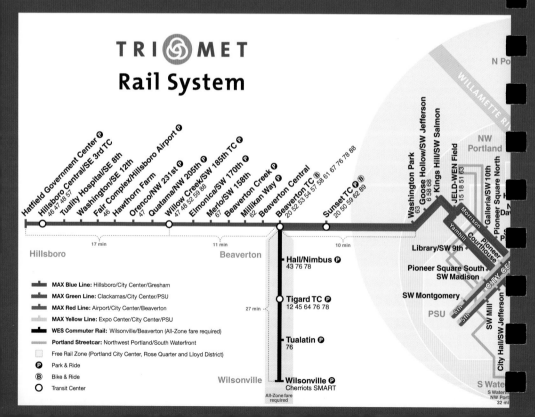

Hatfield Government Center ℗
Hillsboro Central/SE 3rd TC
46 47 48 57
Tuality Hospital/SE 8th
Washington/SE 12th
Fair Complex/Hillsboro Airport ℗
46
Hawthorn Farm
Orenco/NW 231st ℗
47
Quatama/NW 205th ℗
47 48 52 59 88
Willow Creek/SW 185th TC ℗
Elmonica/SW 170th ℗
67
Merlo/SW 158th
Millikan Way ℗
62
Beaverton Creek ℗
Beaverton Central
Beaverton TC ⓑ ℗
20 52 53 54 57 58 61 67 76 78 88
Sunset TC ℗ ⓑ
20 50 59 62 89

Washington Park
63
Goose Hollow/SW Jefferson
6 58 68
Kings Hill/SW Salmon
JELD-WEN Field
15 18 51 63
Galleria/SW 10th
Pioneer Square North
Morrison
Yamhill
Courthouse
Library/SW 9th
Pioneer Square South
SW Madison
SW Montgomery
SW Mill
City Hall/SW Jefferson
5th
6th
PSU

N Po

NW
Portland

WILLAMETTE RI

N
Day

P

CITY CE

S Wate
S Waterfr
NW Port
32 mi

Hillsboro

|← 17 min →|← 11 min →|← 10 min →|

Beaverton

Hall/Nimbus ℗
43 76 78

Tigard TC ℗
12 45 64 76 78

27 min

Tualatin ℗
76

Wilsonville ℗
Cherriots SMART

Wilsonville

All-Zone
fare required

- ▬ **MAX Blue Line:** Hillsboro/City Center/Gresham
- ▬ **MAX Green Line:** Clackamas/City Center/PSU
- ▬ **MAX Red Line:** Airport/City Center/Beaverton
- ▬ **MAX Yellow Line:** Expo Center/City Center/PSU
- ▬ **WES Commuter Rail:** Wilsonville/Beaverton (All-Zone fare required)
- ▬ **Portland Streetcar:** Northwest Portland/South Waterfront
- ☐ Free Rail Zone (Portland City Center, Rose Quarter and Lloyd District)
- ℗ Park & Ride
- ⓑ Bike & Ride
- ○ Transit Center

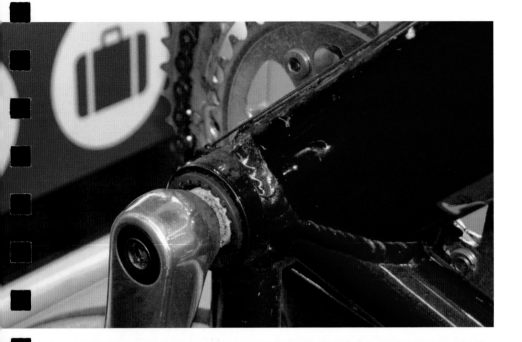

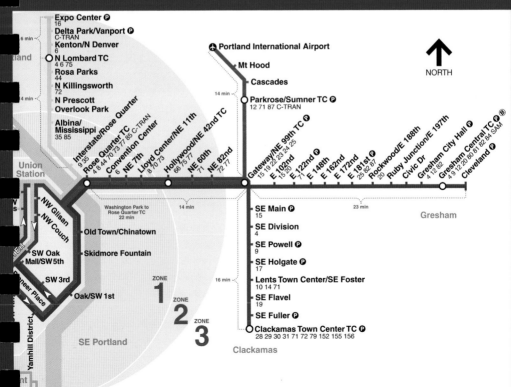

Expo Center P
16

Delta Park/Vanport P
C-TRAN

Kenton/N Denver
6

N Lombard TC
4 6 75

Rosa Parks
44

N Killingsworth
72

N Prescott

Overlook Park

Albina/ Mississippi
35 85

Portland International Airport

Mt Hood

Cascades

Parkrose/Sumner TC P
12 71 87 C-TRAN

NORTH

6 min

land

4 min

14 min

Union Station

Interstate/Rose Quarter

Rose Quarter TC C-TRAN
9 35

Convention Center
4 8 44 70 73 77 85 C-TRAN

NE 7th
6

Lloyd Center/NE 11th
8 70 73

Hollywood/NE 42nd TC
66 75 77

NE 60th
71

NE 82nd
72 77

Gateway/NE 99th TC P
15 19 22 23 24 25

E 102nd
19 20

E 122nd P
71 20

E 148th

E 162nd

E 172nd

E 181st P
25 82 87

Rockwood/E 188th
20

Ruby Junction/E 197th

Civic Dr

Gresham City Hall P
4 12 82

Gresham Central TC P ®
4 9 12 80 81 82 84 SAM

Cleveland P

NW Glisan

NW Couch

Old Town/Chinatown

Skidmore Fountain

SW Oak Mall/SW 5th

SW 3rd

Oak/SW 1st

Pioneer Place

Yamhill District

Washington Park to Rose Quarter TC
22 min

14 min

ZONE 1

ZONE 2

ZONE 3

SE Portland

16 min

23 min

Gresham

SE Main P
15

SE Division
4

SE Powell P
9

SE Holgate P
17

Lents Town Center/SE Foster
10 14 71

SE Flavel
19

SE Fuller P

Clackamas Town Center TC P
28 29 30 31 71 72 79 152 155 156

Clackamas

About the Community Cycling Center

The Community Cycling Center is a nonprofit organization founded in 1994 in Northeast Portland, Oregon. Our mission it to broaden access to bicycling and its benefits. Our vision is to build a vibrant community where people of all backgrounds use bicycles to stay healthy and connected.

In the Beginning

The Community Cycling Center started as a bicycle riding and repair school for kids when founder Brian Lacy noticed kids riding on broken bikes. A trained mechanic, he had an idea: show kids how to fix their bikes and encourage them to try it themselves next time. Then use the fixed bikes to explore the neighborhood, meet neighbors, and learn the history of the area. The concept really came alive when people donated bikes they no longer needed to help those who needed them. In this way, the bicycle became a tool for empowerment.

Where We Are Now

Over time and with the creative contributions of many community-minded people, the Community Cycling Center has grown into a robust nonprofit. We operate a bike shop that specializes in used and refurbished bicycles and helps new riders build their skills and confidence. While we promote safe riding for all, we recognize that the benefits of bicycling are not equally accessible, so we prioritize programs and projects that benefit underserved communities that enable kids to ride to school, adults to ride to work, and for lots of people to ride for health. In 2009, we completed a needs assessment, Understanding Barriers to Bicycling, which provided the foundation for community collaborations where we work closely with community partners to develop programs and projects that overcome barriers. In this way, the bicycle is a vehicle for community change.

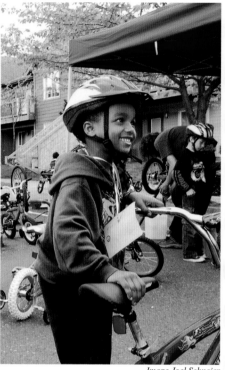

Image Joel Schneier

Where We Are Headed

We believe that all Portlanders, regardless of their income, education or ethnic background, should have the opportunity to choose healthy, active transportation allowing them to live a long, healthy life. So we will be working to make bicycles accessible to get to work or school, spend time with friends or family, or simply explore the city. We will work collaboratively with community partners to overcome barriers to bicycling while building community capacity. We will look at ways to create pathways to employment and engagement within the growing bicycle movement, including jobs as educators, advocates, and mechanics. We will do this so that the promise of a healthy, sustainable Portland is possible for all of its residents.

Expert training, nutrition and technical information in the palm of your hand!

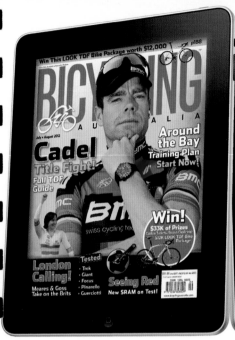

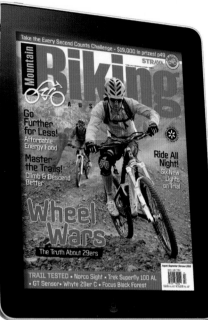

Bicycling Australia is packed with interesting and useful information that will enhance your cycling experience. Our expert writers specialize in providing detailed information on training, positioning, health and nutrition, designed to help you ride better. There's also unbiased, critical analysis of new products—from parts, and accessories, to clothing and nutrition, to full bike reviews—all with detailed photography to help you buy better. You'll also find Where to Ride suggestions in every issue, for destinations both in Australia and overseas. Download your copy now!

Mountain Biking Australia is 'the' magazine for enduro, trail-riding and cross-country mountain bikers. Written by experienced riders who know what they're on about, Mountain Biking Australia features detailed, critical analysis of new bikes, parts, clothing and nutrition. The five in-depth bike tests in each issue give great insight beyond the manufacturers' marketing spin. Brilliant photography gets you up close and personal with the all new gear. There are mechanical 'how-to' tips to help you maintain your gear, and technical riding pointers to help you ride better. A great read for MTBers the world over. Download your copy now!

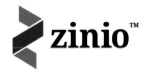

www.bicyclingaustralia.com.au/digital

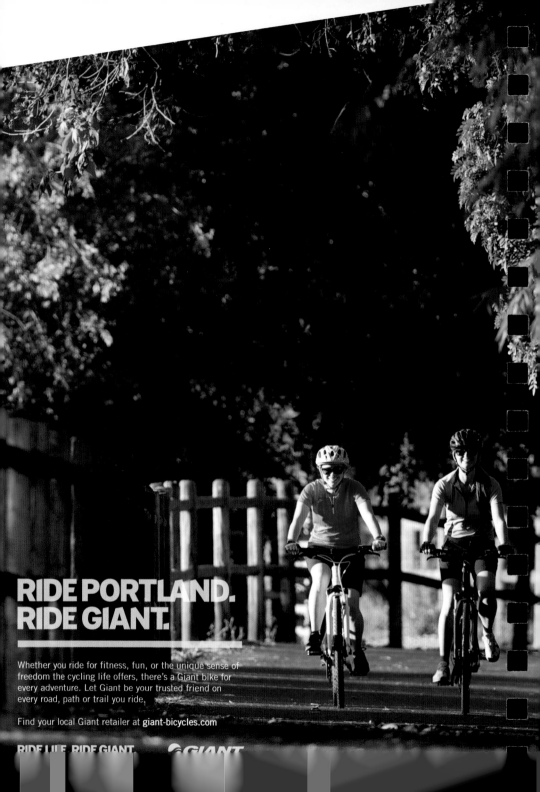

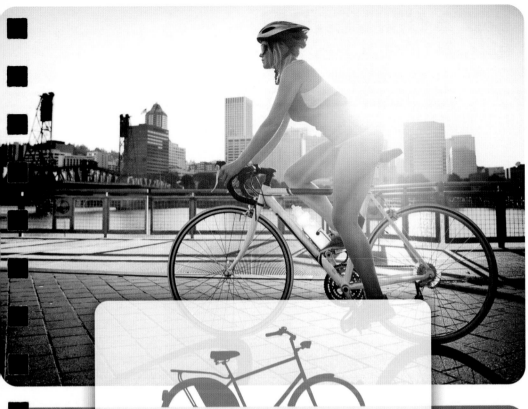

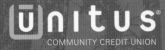

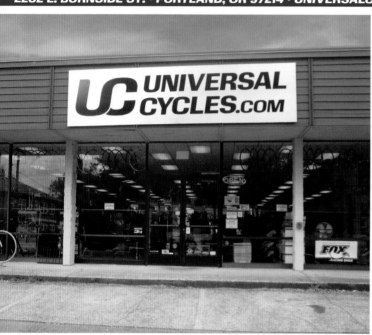
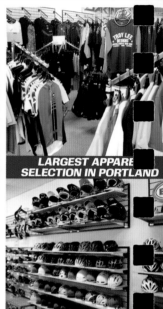
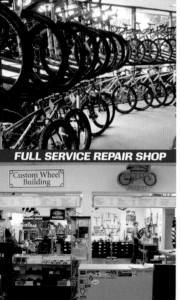
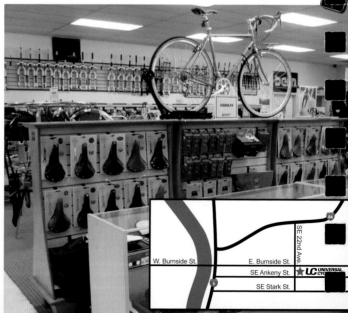

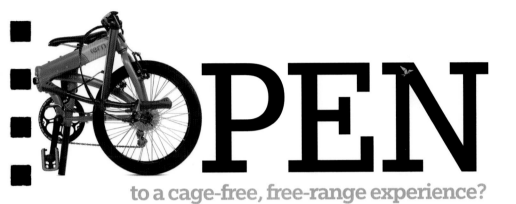

OPEN

to a cage-free, free-range experience?

ternbicycles.com/us

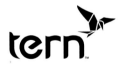

tern™

Where to Bike

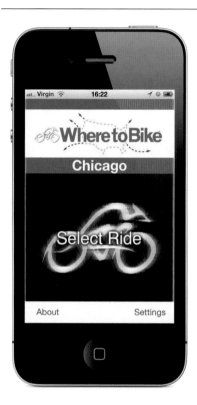

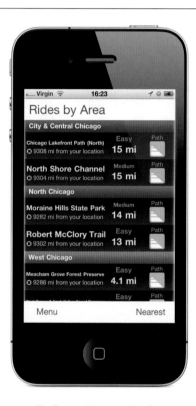

Getting Started

Step 1. Download the *Where to Bike* app for your city on the iTunes App Store. Once you load the app, you'll see this main page where you can select your ride, learn more about us, or configure settings. In the settings menu you can choose between miles and km, whether you want to display your speed, and whether you'd like a fixed or rotating map.

Select Your Ride

Step 2. Tap 'select ride' from the main screen and you will arrive at this page, where you will see a list of great rides organized into sections. These are the same as you will find in your *Where to Bike* book guide. In the bottom right-hand corner you will also see an option to arrange the rides based on their proximity to your current location.

www.**where**to**bike**guides**.com**

Our *Where to Bike* apps are the perfect companion for your next ride. Don't leave home without it!

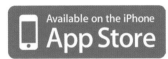 **+** **=**

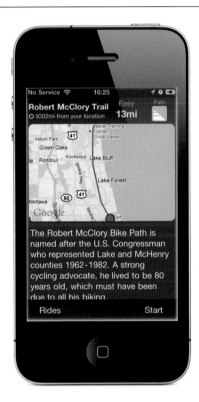

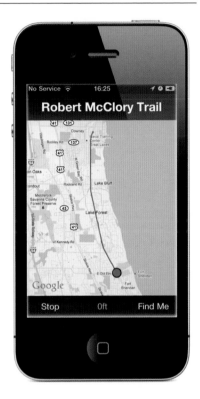

Ride Overview

Step 3. Once you select a ride, you'll be taken to this ride overview screen. Here you'll see a thumbnail map of the route, and a short description of the ride. You will also see important information such as ride difficulty, total distance, as well as how far you currently are from start of the ride. When you are ready, tap the 'Start' button to commence the ride.

Ready to Ride

Step 4. Now you are ready to ride, it really is that simple! Your current position will be displayed by the red dot icon. You can slide your finger to scroll anywhere on the map, and if you lose your place, simply tap 'Find Me' to return to the ride route. If you feel like taking a break, simply tap the 'stop' button and you can continue again whenever you like. Have fun!

North/Northeast

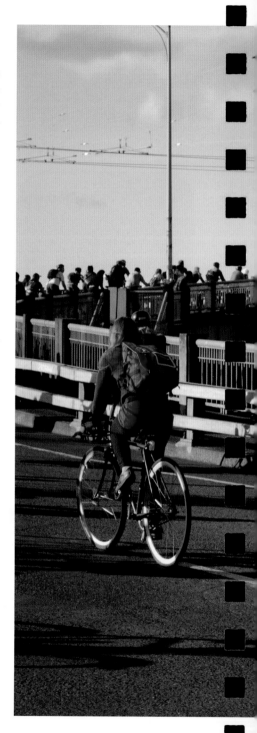

Traversing Oregon and Washington states these rides cover both rural and urban settings. Ride north to the most distant point where you'll find the Ridgefield Wildlife Refuge, explore the areas around the mighty Columbia River, and discover urban treasures in both Vancouver and Portland. While the better part of these rides are fairly flat, you will find yourself challenged with some hills as you go further north. This section contains both the longest ride in the book and the shortest providing the gamut of choices for cyclists of every skill level.

The contrast between the bicycle infrastructure in Portland and Vancouver will be quite apparent to anyone who chooses rides in this section. In Vancouver you will find far fewer cyclists than you encounter in and around Portland. There is plenty of adventure and beautiful sites worthy of your attention in both states, however, and I invite you to explore with enthusiasm. Vancouver is loaded to the brim with a rich history of the early pioneers just waiting for your exploration. Few streets outside of downtown Vancouver have bike lanes, but these rides were designed to provide low-traffic routes for safe cycling. Many of the Vancouver area rides included here are popular with cyclists from both states.

The two bridges crossing the Columbia River each offers a unique adventure. The I-5 Bridge will bring you 80 feet above the water and provides a great view. The I-205 Bridge is part of a bike path that extends from Vancouver in the north to Clackamas Town Center some 20 miles south. Both bridges are exciting in their own special way and worth the experience.

History, nature, and art characterize most of the rides in this section. If you are a bird-watching enthusiast or have just a casual interest, you cannot help but be impressed with the variety of birds you will find around Sauvie Island, at the Wildlife Refuge, and at Smith and Bybee lakes. Spin your way through pioneer history and modern day art as you enjoy the northern reaches of these rides around greater Portland and Vancouver.

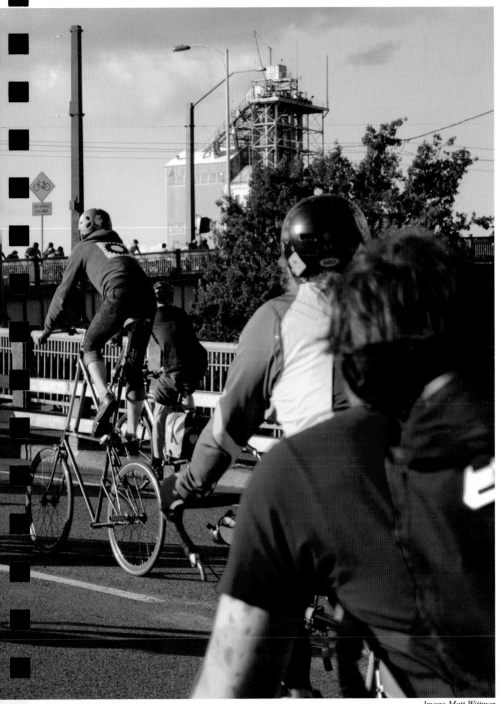

Image Matt Wittmer

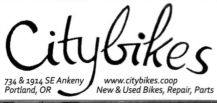
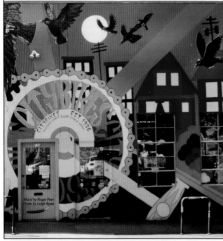
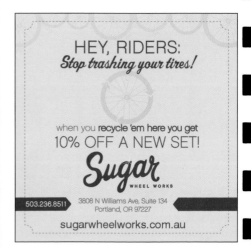
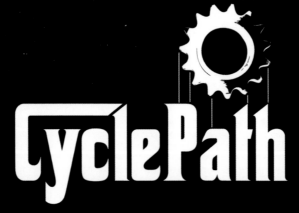

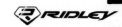

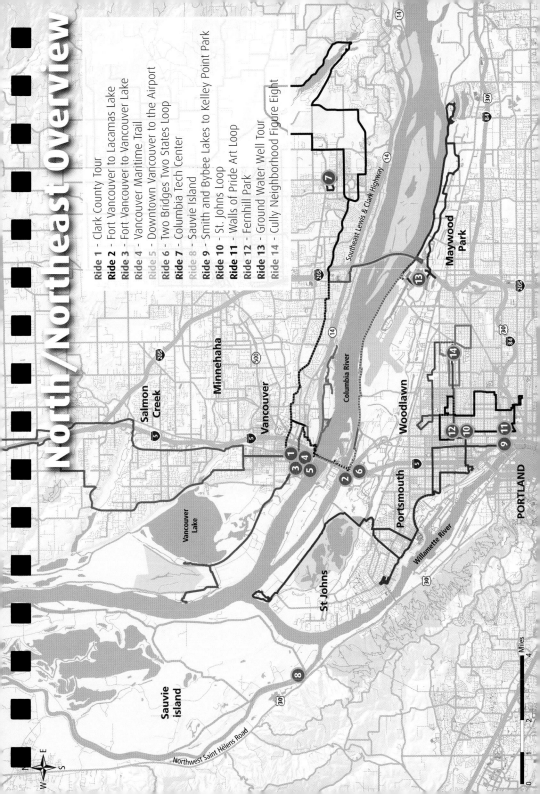

North/Northeast Overview

Ride 1 - Clark County Tour
Ride 2 - Fort Vancouver to Lacamas Lake
Ride 3 - Fort Vancouver to Vancouver Lake
Ride 4 - Vancouver Maritime Trail
Ride 5 - Downtown Vancouver to the Airport
Ride 6 - Two Bridges Two States Loop
Ride 7 - Columbia Tech Center
Ride 8 - Sauvie Island
Ride 9 - Smith and Bybee Lakes to Kelley Point Park
Ride 10 - St. Johns Loop
Ride 11 - Walls of Pride Art Loop
Ride 12 - Fernhill Park
Ride 13 - Ground Water Well Tour
Ride 14 - Cully Neighborhood Figure Eight

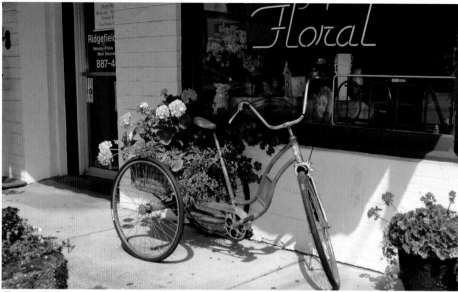

Flowers make this repurposed bicycle beautiful again.

At a Glance

Distance 40.4 miles   **Elevation Gain** 3295'
Distance from Downtown Portland 8.5 miles

Terrain

Smooth paved streets until reaching the Ridgefield National Wildlife Refuge where access roads are rough. Many moderately challenging hills throughout the ride.

Traffic

Low-traffic streets most of the ride with short sections of moderate traffic on wide streets.

How to Get There

By car, take Route I-5 to exit 1B in Vancouver, turn left onto E Sixth Street. On-street parking.

By public transportation, from downtown Portland take Bus #6 to Jantzen Beach Transit Center, transfer to Bus #4 Fourth Plain Eastbound to Broadway and Seventh Street.

Food and Drink

Plenty of options for food and drinks at the starting point of the ride in downtown Vancouver. Restrooms available in Esther Short Park and again at Ridgefield National Wildlife Refuge.

Side Trip

Pearson Air Field Museum and Fort Vancouver are located within riding distance of downtown Vancouver.

Links to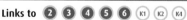

Where to Bike Rating

About...

Begin the ride at beautiful Esther Short Park in downtown Vancouver where there is a vibrant weekend farmers' market, then ride through quiet residential streets to the outskirts of town. Riding through quaint downtown Ridgefield will bring back memories of small town America. Just before reaching Ridgefield, you will thank yourself for taking some time to explore the Ridgefield National Wildlife Refuge. Plan to make this ride a full day excursion to take advantage of all the sights along the route.

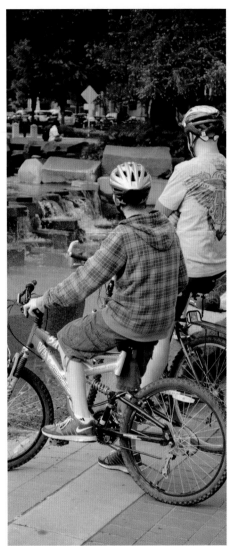

Resting alongside Lazy River at Esther Shore Park.
Image Matt Wittmer

Riding north along wide Columbia Street you will quickly find yourself in residential neighborhoods leaving behind the bustle of downtown Vancouver. The hills begin once you reach about the three mile mark and are peppered throughout the ride. Also abundant on this ride are blackberry bushes, which are full of ripe, juicy fruit in late August.

At about the 15 mile mark along NW Carty Road, you will find the most challenging hill of the ride. The vista of the distant mountains that greets you is well worth the huffing and puffing required to reach the summit. On a clear day you'll have many scenic backdrops to choose from for capturing photos of your ride. While this peak is the highest of the ride, there are plenty of less challenging hills along this route.

The Ridgefield National Wildlife Refuge is a perfect place to enjoy a picnic if you brought one along. Lock your bikes at the parking lot as they are not allowed on the refuge grounds. The wet lands area is full of nesting and migrating birds. Signs direct visitors to remain on roadways in order to limit human interference.

Just a short distance beyond is quaint downtown Ridgefield. The small storefronts bring back memories of small towns where everyone knows their neighbor.

If you didn't bring a picnic, there are several restaurants in this small village. Outside of Ridgefield is the Long House, built by Native Americans as a gathering and worship space. A visit will not take very long and is worth spending a little time to explore.

The return trip brings you back into civilization quickly as you ride along bike lanes on busier streets to end your ride in downtown Vancouver.

Ride Log

0.0 Begin at the corner of Columbia St and W Eighth St in downtown Vancouver and ride north on Columbia St.

1.9 Left onto NW 45th St.

2.3 Right onto NW Lincoln Ave.

3.3 Left onto NW Bernie Dr.

3.9 Right onto NW Lakeshore Ave.

6.5 Cross NW 119th St and NW Lakeshore Ave becomes NW 36th Ave which you will continue to follow.

7.8 Right onto NW Bliss Rd.

8.5 Left onto NW 21st Ave.

8.9 Right onto NW 149th St.

9.4 Left onto NW 11th Ave.

10.1 Right onto NW 164th St (becomes NE 164th St).

11.1 Left onto NE 10th Ave.

11.9 Right onto NE 179th St.

12.0 Left onto NE Delfel Rd.

13.6 Left onto NW 209th St.

14.0 Right onto NW 11th Ave.

15.2 Left onto NW Eklund Rd.

15.5 Left onto NW Carty Rd.

16.7 Right onto NW Hillhurst Rd (becomes S Ninth Ave at Cemetery Rd). Cemetery Rd is at 18.8 miles.

19.1 Left onto Pioneer St.

19.4 Right onto N Main Ave.

20.5 Left to enter the Ridgefield National Wildlife Refuge. Have a rest then turn around.

21.0 Right onto N Main Ave.

21.8 Left onto Pioneer St.

22.1 Right onto S Ninth Ave (aka S Hillhurst Rd).

24.5 Left onto NW Carty Rd.

26.9 Right onto NE 10th Ave.

30.0 Left onto NE 179th St.

30.3 Right onto NE 15th Ave (also known as NE Union Rd).

31.7 Continue straight. At the junction of NE 154th and NE 155th streets, NE Union Rd becomes NE 20th Ave.

32.7 Continue straight. At the intersection of NW 134th St NE 20th Ave becomes NE Hwy 99 (also known as Pacific Hwy).

33.6 Right onto NE 117th St.

34.4 Left onto NE Hazel Dell Ave.

38.0 Right onto E 45th St (becomes NW 45th St).

38.3 Left onto NW Columbia St.

40.4 Return to the corner of Columbia St and W Eighth St. End ride.

 P1 Ridgefield National Wildlife Refuge
P2 Native American Plankhouse

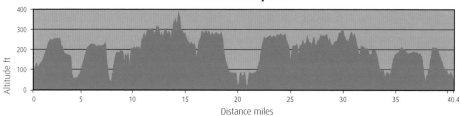

Clark County Tour

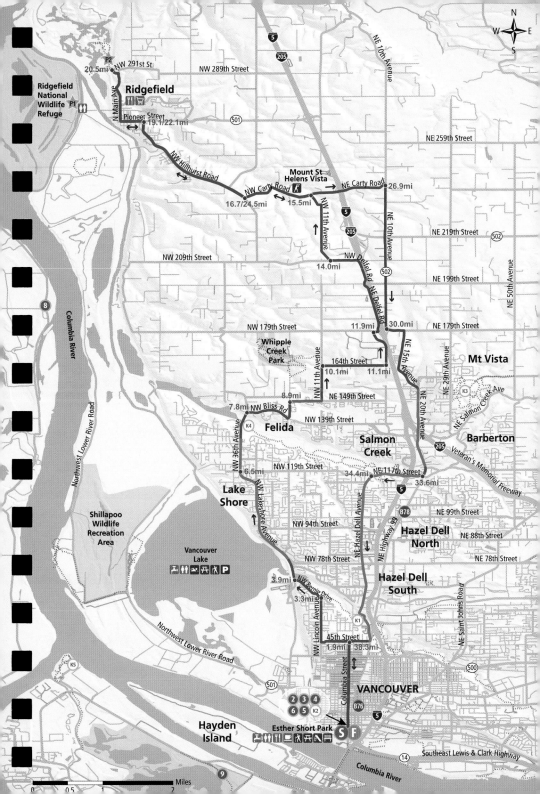

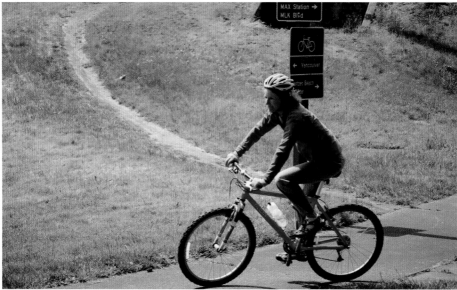

Directional signs mark the way near the I-5 Bridge.   Image Matt Wittmer

At a Glance

Distance 40.4 miles   **Elevation Gain** 1440′
Distance from Downtown Portland 6.9 miles

Terrain

Smooth well-maintained streets, some narrow with no shoulder or bike lane.

Traffic

Low-traffic streets with most intersections having crossing lights.

How to Get There

By car, take I-5 north toward Seattle; take exit 307 for Oregon 99E/Marine Drive toward Delta Park; keep left at the fork, follow signs for M.L.K. Jr Boulevard/ Marine Drive W; turn right onto Marine Drive W. Expo Center is on the left; parking available at the top of N Force Avenue or on-street.

     By public transportation, take the TriMet MAX Yellow line north to the Expo MAX station, the last station.

Food and Drink

There are restrooms and drinking fountains at Esther Short Park and at the far end of Lacamas Lake on NW Lake Road at Camas Heritage Park, and restrooms at the trailhead of the Lacamas Heritage Trail. At the corner of N Devine Road and McArthur Boulevard is River Maiden Artisan Coffee, a café where bicyclists are known to gather.

Side Trips

Visit Fort Vancouver, Pearson Air Museum, Vancouver Library, Green Mountain Golf Course, and Esther Short Park.

Links to   ① ③ ④ ⑤ ⑥ ⑦ ㊹ Ⓚ②

Where to Bike Rating   🚲🚲🚲🚲

About...

From the last train station of the yellow TriMet MAX line, cross the expansive Columbia River via the I-5 Bridge 80 feet above the river and descend into downtown Vancouver. Then travel east through quiet residential neighborhoods. Loop around picturesque Lacamas Lake before returning to downtown Vancouver. Along the way you'll enjoy traveling through historic Fort Vancouver along Officers Row.

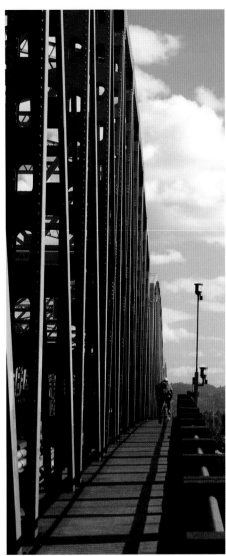

Spanning the Columbia with space aplenty.
Image Matt Wittmer

Starting at the busy intersection of N Marine Drive you'll access the bike path that will bring you across the Columbia River. On a warm summer day, 80 feet above the river, you'll have a vista of sailboats, power boats, ships and tankers, but pay attention as the path is narrow. You'll descend into downtown Vancouver and head east through residential neighborhoods that eventually dissolve to rural farmland.

Crossing into the town of Camas traveling along the ridge above the lake, you can catch glimpses of the lake between the houses on your left. As you come around to the far side of the lake, the road narrows considerably, but there is little traffic to hinder your ride. If you make this trip in late summer, you'll be rewarded with an abundance of ripe, sweet blackberries growing along the side of the road. Lacamas Lake is popular for fishing and boating. On the day of our ride there were great expanses of water lilies at the far end of the lake ready to bloom.

On the return trip, after turning onto NE 28th Street, the traffic speeds up a bit, but the road is wider here as you travel past the golf course and farms. At 192nd Street you'll see way-finding signs for Fisher's Landing and downtown Vancouver, and you'll pick up a bike lane that is considerably wider.

Descend the hill to enter Fort Vancouver through the stockade fence and enjoy the slow pace of riding through the fort apple orchard. Ride over the land bridge down to the Oldest Apple Tree park, under the railroad bridge, and you will quickly find yourself back in an urban setting. Crossing the Columbia River will be easier traveling south as the pathway is a little wider.

Ride Log

- P1 Fort Vancouver & Pearson Air Museum
- P2 Officer's Row
- P3 Oldest Apple Tree
- P4 Lacamas Heritage Trail
- P5 River Maiden Artisen Coffee

0.0 From Expo MAX Station, ride up to N Marine Dr; right onto sidewalk.

0.1 Left to cross N Marine Dr; access bike path on opposite side.

0.4 Left at sign for Marine Dr Vancouver; right through tunnel; ride parallel with I-5 to rotary; cross intersection via the pedestrian crossing to stay straight; remain on sidewalk; cross next intersection with pedestrian crossing to take left and access bike path. Left upon crossing, ride parallel to I-5 and cross bridge.

2.1 Right onto Columbia St.

3.1 Right onto McLoughlin Blvd.

5.4 Right onto Brandt Rd.

5.5 Left onto E Mill Plain Blvd.

5.9 Right onto McArthur Blvd.

7.8 Dog leg right onto St. Helens Rd.

8.5 Right onto SE 98th Ave.

8.6 Left onto SE 10th St (becomes SE McGillivray Blvd).

11.9 Right onto SE Village Loop (becomes SE 29th St).

13.0 Right onto SE 176th St.

13.2 Left onto SE 34th St (becomes Pacific Rim Blvd).

15.3 Left onto NW Parker St.

16.8 Right onto NW Lake Rd.

19.3 Left onto NE Everett St.

19.9 Left onto SE Leadbetter Rd, then right into NE 232nd Ave.

22.8 Left onto NE 28th St, then left into NW Friberg-Strunk St.

25.4 Right onto SE First St.

25.9 Left onto 192nd St.

26.9 Right onto SE 20th St.

28.5 Right onto SE McGillivray Blvd.

31.8 Right onto SE 98th Ave.

31.9 Left onto St. Helens Ave.

32.6 Dog leg right onto McArthur Blvd.

34.5 Left onto E Mill Plain Blvd.

35.0 Right onto Brandt Rd; left onto McLoughlin Blvd.

36.2 Left onto E Reserve St.

36.6 Right onto E Evergreen Blvd.

36.8 Left into Fort Vancouver. Right onto E Fifth St; enter fort via bike pathway to access land bridge.

37.9 Right onto SE Columbia Way.

38.1 Right onto I-5 bike path; cross bridge; follow path to right; follow sign for bike route through tunnel; left at end of tunnel; cross street with pedestrian crossing light.

39.2 Right onto access road sidewalk; cross intersection; access sidewalk on opposite side; follow bike path to left; follow signs to Marine Dr West.

39.7 Right toward Marine Dr West; notice road signs for Expo Center and Marine Dr ahead.

40.3 Right onto opposite sidewalk at N Marine Dr.

40.4 Ride to Expo MAX Station. End ride.

Fort Vancouver to Lacamas Lake

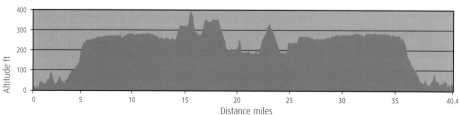

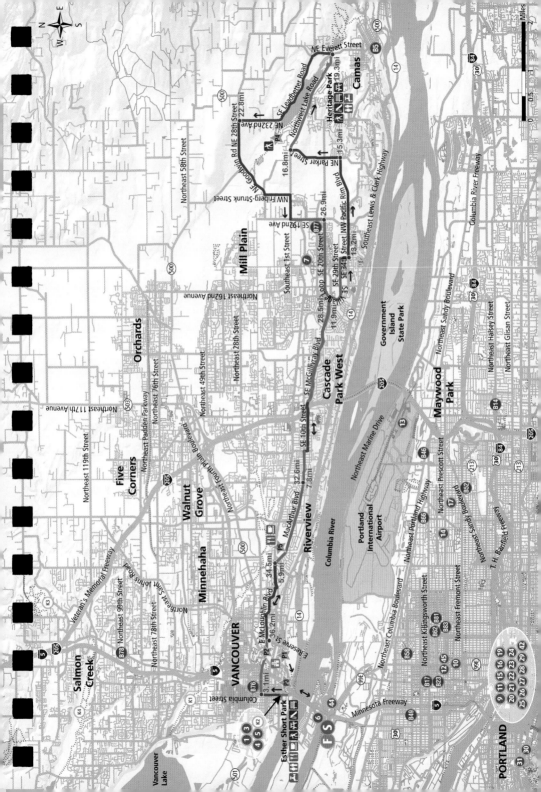

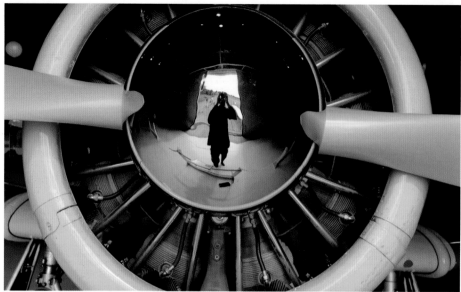

Up close and personal at the Pearson Air Museum.   *Image Matt Wittmer*

At a Glance

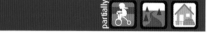

Distance 18.8 miles   **Elevation Gain** 306'

Distance from Downtown Portland 8.5 miles

Terrain

Smooth, well-maintained streets with a short section of hard-packed gravel.

Traffic

Low-traffic streets with most intersections having crossing lights.

How to Get There

By car, take Route I-5 north toward Seattle. After crossing the I-5 Bridge, take the second exit and follow signs to City Center. On-street parking.

   By public transportation, from downtown Portland take Bus #6 to Jantzen Beach Transit Center, transfer to Bus #4 Fourth Plain Eastbound to Broadway and Seventh Street.

Food and Drink

There are restrooms and drinking fountains at Esther Short Park, Vancouver Lake, and at the end of Fisherman's Bar Trail. Food and restaurants can be found in downtown Vancouver.

Side Trips

Visit the parks along the route, the Pearson Air Museum, Fort Vancouver, Vancouver Library, and the railroad yard along Evergreen.

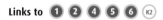

Links to ① ② ④ ⑤ ⑥ (K2)

Where to Bike Rating

About...

This ride brings you through the historic sites of Vancouver to present day deep-water Port Vancouver. Begin by visiting historic Fort Vancouver and the Pearson Air Museum and travel along the street of carefully preserved houses of Officer's Row. You'll leave this behind and ride through the modern-day inter-modal area of Port Vancouver and come to the confluence of the Multnomah Channel and Columbia River where oil tankers await entry to port.

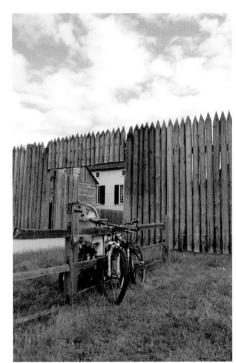

A family of bicycles outside the Fort Vancouver palisade.
Image Matt Wittmer

Begin at Propstra Square in Esther Short Park under the Glockenspiel and ride south toward the bridge. You will quickly come to the entrance to Fort Vancouver where you'll find the carefully maintained Oldest Apple Tree in the northwest. The land bridge will bring you through history with photos and vista points until you reach Fort Vancouver. Established in 1824, Fort Vancouver was a fur trading outpost and headquarters of the Hudson Bay Company. The current buildings are replicas of the originals which were destroyed in a fire.

Pearson Air Museum is located a short distance from the fort. The museum specializes in airplanes built during or prior to World War II. The museum has one-of-a-kind aircraft on display in one of the oldest wooden hangars in the U.S.

Part of the National Historic site is an expanse of fields with picnic tables, a gazebo, and play structures. This fort is the site of one of the largest Independence Day fireworks displays west of the Mississippi River. Exiting the fort you will ride along Officer's Row under a mature tree canopy that not only provides welcome shade on a hot summer day, but also frames the magnificent houses, one of which was constructed for Ulysses S. Grant.

As you leave the fort area, you will ride through downtown Vancouver heading toward Vancouver Lake. This wonderful park has a beach, picnic shelters and is a popular place for boating and kayaking. There are a number of play structures and plenty of open space for a quick game of softball.

Leaving the lake, you'll travel along the Frenchman's Bar Trail through farmland. This area is directly across from Sauvie Island where the Multnomah Channel and the Columbia River come together. Ships access Port Vancouver here and it is common to see several enormous tankers awaiting entry to port. Cyclists can enter the park at no cost via the bike path.

On your return trip, stop on the bridge above the railroad yard and you're sure to see a train or two loaded with goods. Esther Short Park is the perfect place to end this ride. Here you'll be able to enjoy a picnic, visit the farmers market, or just sit in one of the local cafés with your favorite beverage.

Ride Log

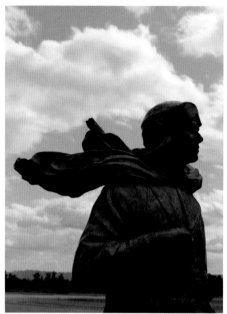

Carlton F. Bond, commanding officer, 121st Squadron, Army Air Corps. Image Matt Wittmer

 P1 Oldest Apple Tree
P2 Fort Vancouver National Historic Site
P3 Pearson Air Museum
P4 Officer's Row
P5 Vancouver Library
P6 Railroad juncture

2.5 Right onto Columbia St.

2.7 Left onto W 15th St which becomes W Mill Plain Blvd and then becomes W Fourth Plain Blvd for a short distance before becoming NW Lower River Rd.

7.4 Right into Vancouver Lake.

8.1 Reverse direction and ride via the same path to return to the park entrance.

8.9 Left to the opposite side of the road.

9.0 Right to ride along the Frenchman's Bar Trail which parallels NW Lower River Rd.

10.8 Left to enter Frenchman's Bar via the bike path.

11.3 Reverse direction at the end of the bike path and return to the park entrance.

11.8 Right onto Frenchman's Bar Trail.

13.7 Right onto NW Lower River Rd to return along the same road to downtown Vancouver.

17.4 After crossing over Thompson Rd, access sidewalk to cross the bridge; railroad tracks below.

18.0 Return to the bike lane in the street along W 15th St.

18.3 Right at the fork onto one-way section of W 15th St.

18.4 Right onto Columbia St.

18.8 Return to corner of Columbia and E Sixth streets. End ride.

0.0 Begin at Esther Short Park, at the corner of Columbia and E Sixth streets. Ride south under the I-5 Bridge either on the wide street or on the sidewalk.

0.5 Left under railroad bridge at sign for Fort Vancouver National Site. Ride through Fort Vancouver.

1.1 Right at the end of the path onto E Fifth St.

1.2 Left into the park entrance and ride up the hill.

1.6 Left at the stop sign onto Evergreen Blvd and ride along Officer's Row; ride through roundabout staying on Evergreen.

Fort Vancouver to Vancouver Lake

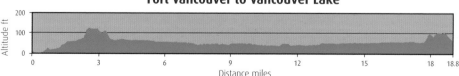

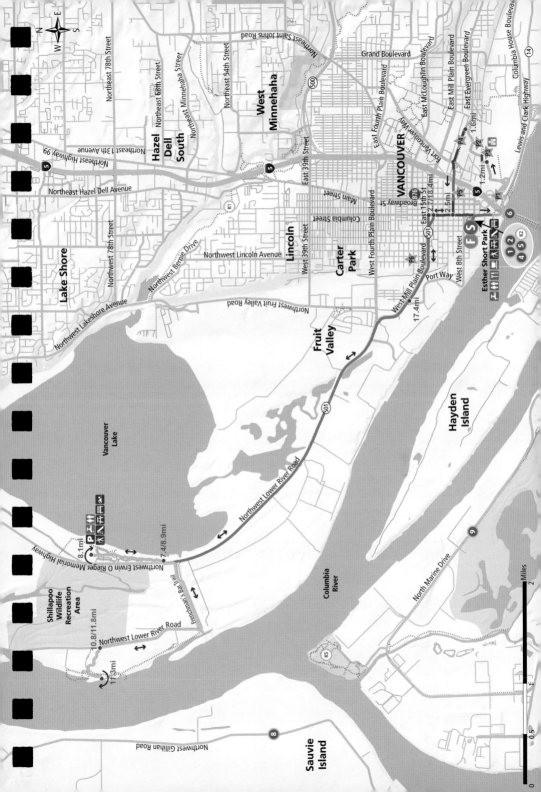

Vancouver Maritime Trail Ride 4

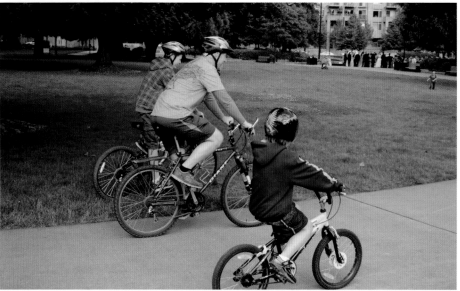

This ride begins and ends in the oldest public square in Washington. Image Matt Wittmer

At a Glance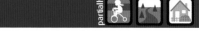

Distance 11.6 miles   **Elevation Gain** 425′
Distance from Downtown Portland 8.5 miles

Terrain

Smooth, paved streets and bike/pedestrian paths.

Traffic

Paved bike/pedestrian paths on most of this ride. Urban streets have low to moderate traffic with bike lanes.

How to Get There

By car, take I-5 to exit 1B in Vancouver, turn left onto E Sixth Street. On-street parking.

By public transportation, from downtown Portland take Bus #6 to Jantzen Beach Transit Center, transfer to Bus #4 Fourth Plain Eastbound to Broadway and Seventh Street.

Food and Drink

Plenty of options for food and drinks at the starting point of the ride in downtown Vancouver. Restrooms available in Esther Short Park, at the parks along the ride, and at the visitor center of Fort Vancouver.

Side Trip

Pearson Air Field Museum is located along the route.

Links to ① ② ③ ⑤ ⑥ (K2)

Where to Bike Rating

About...

The rich maritime history of Vancouver is part of the fun of this ride. You'll enjoy views of the Columbia River tucked behind rows of storefronts and condominiums before riding to the far end of the trail where the expanse of the river at Marine Park can be seen from the lookout tower and then again at Wintler Community Park from the edge of the shore. You'll enjoy more of the area's history riding through Fort Vancouver.

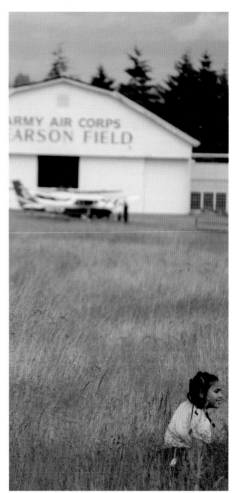

Lazing on Fort Vancouver's lovely grounds.
Image Matt Wittmer

Begin at Propstra Square in Esther Short Park on the corner of W Sixth Avenue and Columbia Street, and ride south toward the I-5 Bridge. After riding under the railroad trestle you can pick up the wide bike/pedestrian pathway just before reaching the I-5 Bridge. There will be plenty of cyclists and pedestrians along the path, but be particularly careful of the children who especially like to ride their bikes here.

The bike path splits with the wider section continuing straight. Take the right fork to ride behind the buildings along the river. This path is not used frequently and you may have this section completely to yourself. The view of the river along here is terrific. While the area is secluded, it is only one block from the shops along SE Columbia Way.

Leave this pathway and return to SE Columbia Way to continue on your journey to Marine Park. If you do this ride on a weekend you'll find very little traffic as this is an industrial area which is quiet on non-business days. Marine Park has a popular boat launch and a lookout tower.

Returning along SE Columbia Way, you'll access Fort Vancouver via the land bridge to cross the highway. Doing so will take you back in history to the earliest days of Vancouver. Just beyond the fort you'll find the Pearson Air Museum which is worth a visit. Fort Vancouver has a wonderful, hilly field where you'll find picnic tables to enjoy a break. The visitor center at the fort will provide you with plenty of historical information about the area.

Continue your ride along shady Officer's Row where the U.S. Grant House is located. After the roundabout you will find yourself on a busier urban street that takes you back to Columbia Street and your starting point.

Ride Log

P1 Oldest Apple Tree
P2 Fort Vancouver National Historic Site
P3 Pearson Air Museum
P4 Officer's Row
P5 Vancouver Library

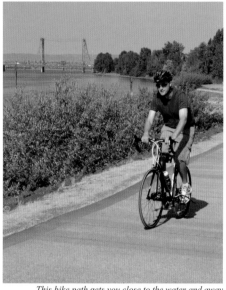

This bike path gets you close to the water and away from traffic.

0.0 Begin at the corner of W Sixth St and Columbia St in downtown Vancouver and ride south.

0.2 Continue straight under railroad trestle. Columbia St is also known as SE Columbia Way from this point.

1.1 Right onto bike path that follows the river.

1.6 Reverse direction and continue along bike path.

1.7 Right turn between buildings onto perpendicular bike path.

1.8 Right turn to ride along street side of buildings.

1.9 Left along bike path back to SE Columbia Way.

2.0 Right onto SE Columbia Way.

3.1 Right onto SE Marine Park Way.

3.6 Reverse direction and return along SE Marine Park Way.

4.0 Right onto bike path through Marine Park.

4.2 Right onto SE Columbia Way.

5.0 Right through parking lot to access bike path along the river.

5.1 Left to follow bike path to Wintler Park.

5.5 Reverse direction.

6.0 Right at the parking lot; left onto SE Columbia Way.

9.1 Right onto bike path under railroad trestle at Fort Vancouver.

9.2 Right onto land bridge pathway. Follow path over highway and through Fort Vancouver.

9.8 Right onto E Fifth St.

10.2 Left onto E Reserve St.

10.3 Left onto E Evergreen Blvd.

10.8 Enter roundabout and exit to continue riding along E Evergreen Blvd.

11.3 Left onto Columbia St.

11.6 Return to the corner of W Sixth St and Columbia St. End ride.

Vancouver Maritime Trail

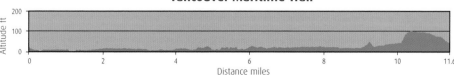

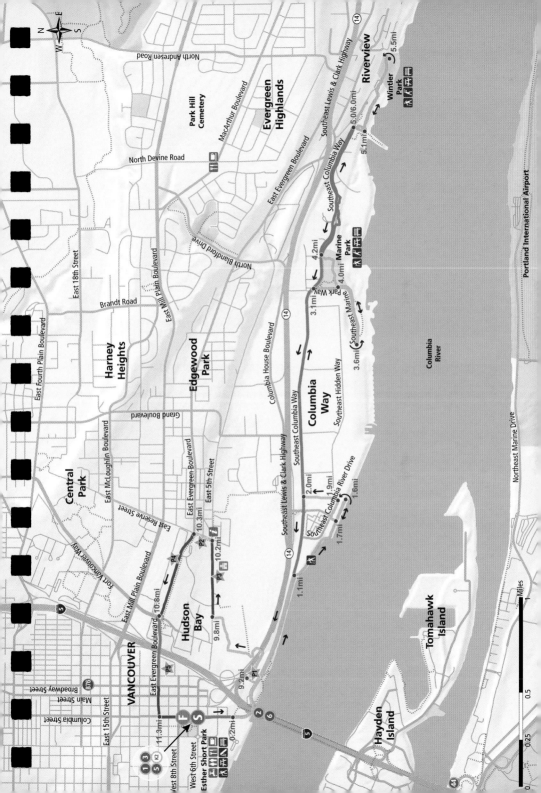

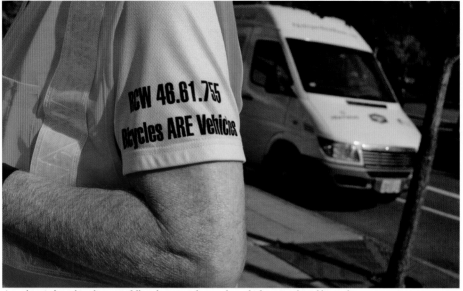

A good reminder ... bicyclists must follow the same rules as other vehicles using the public roads.

At a Glance

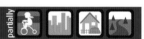

Distance 11.0 miles   **Elevation Gain** 240′
Distance from Downtown Portland 8.5 miles

Terrain

Paved streets and multi-use pathway. Narrow sidewalk/bike path over the Route I-5 Bridge.

Traffic

Urban traffic on streets. Bike paths have low traffic with the exception of the Marine Drive bike path which is low to moderate.

How to Get There

By car, take I-5 north to Seattle; take exit 1B toward City Center/Convention Center; left on E Sixth Street; right onto Columbia Street. On-street parking.

By public transportation, take C-Tran Bus #105 from the corner of SW Sixth Avenue and SW Taylor Street in downtown Portland; disembark at Broadway and Seventh Street in downtown Vancouver.

Food and Drink

Available at the beginning of the ride in downtown Vancouver and again at the Portland airport at the end of the ride.

Side Trip

Explore downtown Vancouver and Esther Short Park; ride the full length of Marine Drive Bike Trail.

Links to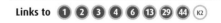

Where to Bike Rating

About...

If you are visiting the greater Portland area, you may want to know how to get to the Portland airport by bicycle. Portland is one of the great places in the world where you can get around exclusively by bike—including riding to and from the airport. This one-way, mostly flat trip provides you with an easy way to travel to/ from the airport from downtown Vancouver, Washington.

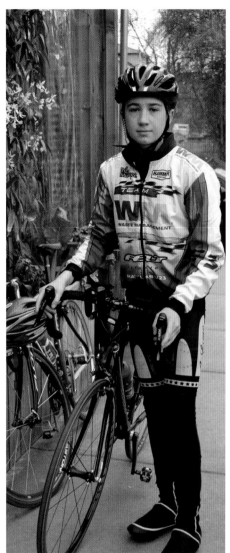

Young cyclists in Portland develop a serious attitude toward cycling.

You can be completely comfortable taking your bike as your sole means of transportation and beginning your adventure the moment you step off the plane. And if you have found another bike-friendly place you would like to visit beyond the Pacific Northwest, you can begin your adventure by riding to the airport using this route.

Some would say that crossing the Columbia River via the I-5 Bridge is a harrowing experience. I would not be one of those people! Though the sidewalk is narrow, it is completely separated from motor traffic. Pedestrians and other cyclists using the same sidewalk are very polite and make way for others. Begin your ride in downtown Vancouver and take the I-5 Bike Path. The bridge will loom ahead of you shortly after you make the left turn off Columbia Street. After crossing the bridge you will be on low-traffic bike paths as you follow I-5 to Marine Drive.

For several miles of this trip you can enjoy the beauty of the Columbia River and watch the airplanes as they take off and land. There is no way to go in the wrong direction – just head toward the airport tower! After crossing over Marine Drive for the second time you may be confused about how to access Frontage Road. Simply follow the bike path and you can't go wrong. Once you arrive at the airport you will be as-tounded at the number of bicycles that are locked up waiting for their owners to return. Whether you decide to ride to the airport and leave your bike behind or take it with you, this is a very pleasant way to meet your flight. The airport even provides a bike stand and tools (located near the TriMet MAX station under the escalator). Enjoy your trip!

Ride Log

0.0 Begin at the corner of W Sixth and Columbia streets in downtown Vancouver and travel south toward the I-5 Bridge to Portland.

0.2 Left onto the I-5 Bike Path immediately after riding under the railroad bridge to cross the I-5 Bridge over the Columbia River.

1.8 Follow the bike path around into the parking lot staying on the sidewalk and ride through the tunnel following signs to Marine Dr.

1.1 Left on the bike path down to the traffic light and cross N Hayden Island Dr. Staying on the sidewalk, cross again with the pedestrian light and ride in the opposite direction of the traffic to access the bike path.

1.8 Ride along the I-5 Bike Path turning left at the sign for Marine Dr into the cul-de-sac of N Anchor Way.

2.4 Left onto N Marine Dr.

4.4 Right onto N 33rd Ave and then left through the underpass to access the bike path.

5.4 Cross N Marine Dr to continue on the opposite side and ride along the dyke.

8.7 Just before the I-205 Bridge follow the signs to the Portland airport riding up the ramp and crossing N Marine Dr.

9.0 Left around NE 96th Ave then right onto NE Airport Way/Frontage Rd.

10.8 Remain on the bike path and ride into the terminal. Continue on the sidewalk to the bike parking.

11.0 End ride.

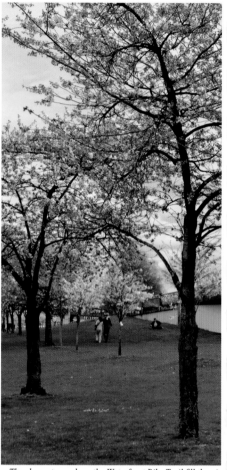

The cherry trees along the Waterfront Bike Trail fill the air with fragrance in early spring.

Downtown Vancouver to the Airport

Altitude ft

Distance miles

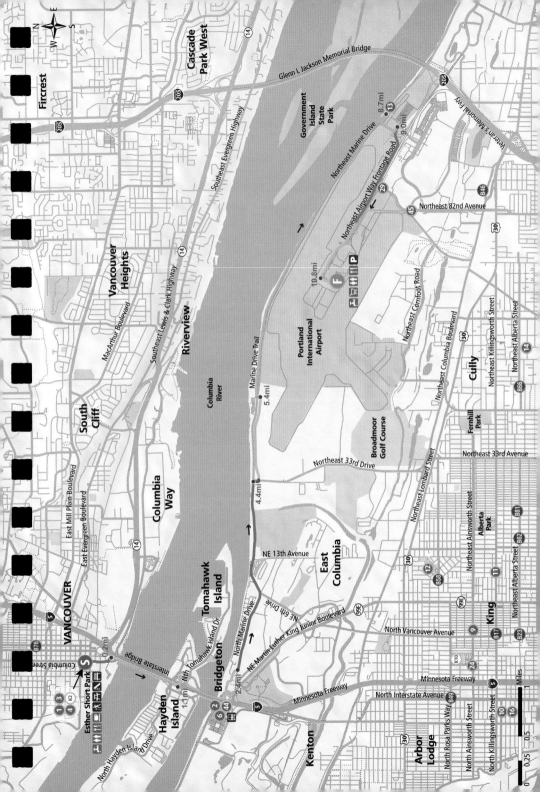

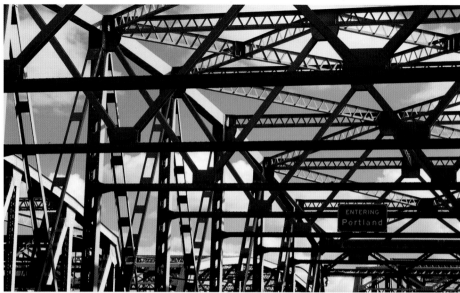

Steel and sky high above the Columbia.

Image Matt Wittmer

At a Glance

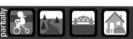

Distance 20.7 miles   **Elevation Gain** 720′

Distance from Downtown Portland 8.5 miles

Terrain

Smooth, paved streets and popular bike/pedestrian paths.

Traffic

Paved bike/pedestrian paths on most of this ride. Urban streets have low to moderate traffic with bike lanes.

How to Get There

By car, take Route I-5 north toward Seattle; take exit 307 for Oregon 99E/Marine Drive toward Delta Park; keep left at the fork, follow signs for M.L.K. Jr Boulevard/Marine Drive W; turn right onto Marine Drive W. Expo Center is on the left; parking available at the top of N Force Avenue or on-street.

By public transportation, take the TriMet MAX yellow line north to the Expo MAX station, the last station.

Food and Drink

There are restaurants along Marine Drive and in Vancouver on the return ride. Restrooms available in Esther Short Park.

Side Trips

Explore downtown Vancouver, stop along Marine Drive to watch the planes take off and land, or visit Blue Lake Regional Park.

Links to ① ② ③ ④ ⑤ ⑬ ㊹ (K2)

Where to Bike Rating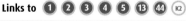

About...

This iconic Portland/Vancouver ride is very popular with local bicycling clubs. It has the intrigue of traveling two states and riding across the two bridges connecting Oregon and Washington states. You'll also ride along cycling paths that parallel two of the most heavily traveled highways without having to tangle with traffic. This is a must ride for anyone who wants to be considered a committed cyclist in the area.

Taking public transportation to the starting point of this ride will prove that getting around Portland without a car is truly possible. Begin by crossing Marine Drive W onto the bike path. Don't miss the sign for Vancouver/ Marine Drive. Take a right and go through the tunnel to ride along the highway onto Hayden Island and then cross the I-5 Bridge.

When you exit, be careful riding through the parking lot to the street. Traffic can be heavy at times, but Vancouver streets are wide and provide ample room for bicycles. There are a couple of tricky turns. The first is after turning onto SE 98th Avenue. Travel halfway down the hill to take the left onto SE 10th Street. The second is on SE 23rd Avenue. You may think you have taken a wrong turn because the street is narrow and dead-ends. Take heart! There is a sign tucked into the woods on the left side of the road that you cannot see until you come to the dead end. It directs you to the bike path and brings you very close to the overpass which is a bit strange, but the real thrill is when you ride up to the middle of the I-205 highway. The traffic travels on both sides and the noise level is high, but the path is separated by fences for a safe ride back to Portland.

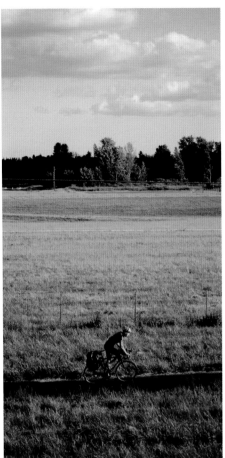

Digging in along Marine Drive. Image Matt Wittmer

Once in Oregon, again access the Marine Drive Trail and ride along the Columbia River. This very popular multi-use path will have plenty of bike and pedestrian traffic on a good day. Just after you cross onto Marine Drive Trail, stop and enjoy the view of Mount Hood behind you. This is also a terrific place to watch the planes landing at the Portland airport. They come directly overhead – quite a sight!

You'll leave Marine Drive when it veers right to ride into the small harbor where you'll be greeted by the sights and sounds of a small marine village complete with marina and houseboats. From here it is a short ride back to your starting point at the Expo MAX station.

Ride Log

0.0 Begin at the Expo TriMet MAX station on the yellow line. Right onto Marine Dr W via the sidewalk to the traffic light. Left to cross Marine Dr W and access the bike path on the opposite side and ride in opposite direction of traffic.

0.4 Left onto bike path at sign for "Vancouver, Marine Drive" and follow path to cross the I-5 Bridge. Take right bike path (a short distance) and ride through the tunnel which goes under the bike path you were just on.

0.7 Cross Columbia Slough into Hayden Island along I-5.

1.1 Continue straight via sidewalk. In order to do this, you must cross N Tomahawk Island Dr via the pedestrian crossing.

1.2 Left at next traffic light onto bike path. Cross via pedestrian traffic signal then left on the bike path to circle around and ride along the bike path next to I-5 and cross Columbia River.

2.1 Right through parking lot then right onto SE Columbia Way (also known as Columbia St).

3.2 Right onto W McLoughlin Blvd (which becomes E McLoughlin Blvd at Main St).

5.5 Right onto Brandt Rd then left onto E Mill Plain Blvd.

5.9 Right onto McArthur Blvd.

7.9 Jog right onto St. Helens Ave.

8.5 Right onto SE 98th Ave.

8.6 Left half way down the hill onto SE 10th St.

9.2 Right onto SE Ellwood Rd.

9.8 Left onto SE 23rd St to end of road.

10.1 Left onto bike path to cross I-205 Bridge (also known as War Veterans Memorial Freeway).

12.7 Left at NE Airport Way.

12.8 Left onto I-205 multi-use path.

13.0 Cross NE Marine Dr to take a left onto Marine Dr Bike Path.

17.1 Bike path ends. Cross NE Marine Dr to access bike path on opposite side.

18.0 Right onto access road along NE 33rd Ave up to Marine Dr.

18.1 Left onto NE Marine Dr.

19.0 Continue onto NE Bridgeton Rd where NE Marine Dr veers left.

19.7 Left onto N Gantenbein Ave.

19.8 Right onto N Marine Dr.

20.1 Right onto N Anchor Way.

20.4 At cul de sac access bike path and turn right.

20.6 Cross Marine Dr W and turn right via sidewalk to ride in the opposite direction of traffic.

20.7 Left onto sidewalk and ride down to Expo Tri-Met station. End ride.

P1 Mount Hood
P2 Blue Lake Regional State Park
P3 Fort Vancouver, Pearson Air Museum
P4 Oldest Apple Tree
P5 River Maiden Artisen Coffee

Two Bridges Two States Loop

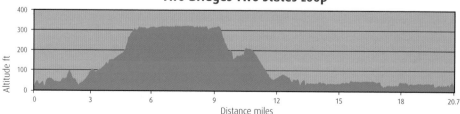

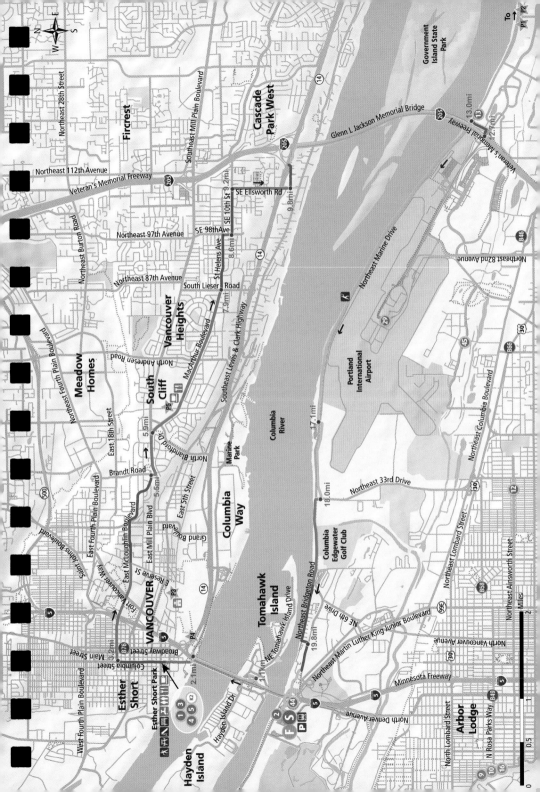

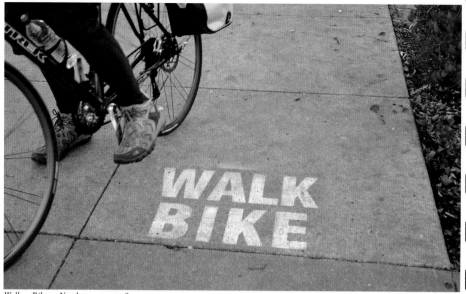

Walk ... Bike ... Need we say more?

At a Glance

Distance 2.95 miles **Elevation Gain** 20′

Distance from Downtown Portland 18.3 miles

Terrain

Smooth, paved streets and bike/pedestrian paths.

Traffic

Paved bike/pedestrian paths and low traffic streets with bike lanes.

How to Get There

By car, take Route I-5 north toward Seattle; take exit 1A for WA-14E toward Camas; take exit 8 for SE 164th Avenue. Turn right onto SE Tech Center Drive then turn right onto SE Sequoia Circle. On-street parking.

Accessing this ride via public transportation is not recommended.

Food and Drink

There are restaurants very close to the boundaries of the Tech Center. The only public restroom is a portable toilet at the softball field.

Side Trips

Lacamas Lake, the Ridgefield Wildlife Refuge and downtown Vancouver are all within a reasonably short drive.

Links to

Where to Bike Rating

About...

This short, flat ride is a perfect way to get familiar with bicycling if you haven't been on a bike for a while. The streets are wide and have well marked bike lanes. On weekends the tech center is very quiet because most of the buildings are active only during business hours. The area is well landscaped with ponds, waterfalls, and a beautiful park that is popular with families and is located next to the Columbia Valley Elementary School.

Plan to drive to the Columbia Tech Center if you are starting from downtown Portland. Public transportation is infrequent to this location. Once you have parked near the Columbia Valley Elementary School, however, you will find others who have discovered this popular area for bicycling and walking. Begin at the park next to the school. There is a slight elevation here, but the rest of the ride is level. Ride through the park where you'll find flat grassy expanses, waterfalls, a duck pond, and lots of benches where you can sit and enjoy the quiet scenery.

Since Columbia Tech Center is an industrial center, there will be very few vehicles on the roads during the weekend. After you leave the park, ride along the tree-lined roads of the center with wide bike lanes. Even though you are on public streets, this is a family-friendly ride since there is virtually no traffic on weekends.

The outlined route brings you past all of the interesting sights. Ride through the park so that you become familiar with your bicycle and gain confidence to ride through the Tech Center streets. Along the way you will find a secluded softball field tucked behind some of the buildings. This is where the only public restroom is located.

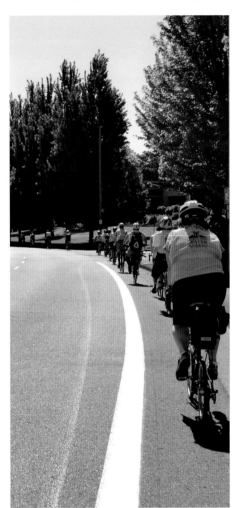

The roads through the industrial park have wide lanes and low weekend traffic.

The Tech Center is surrounded by the wide bustling streets of suburban Vancouver, and on one corner of the industrial park is a shopping center with plenty of restaurant choices if you decided not to bring a picnic. Since the route is flat you may want to make the loop a couple of times. There is plenty to see and the park is a terrific place to bring children. They can play in the field, watch the ducks in the pond, and have a picnic. With small children the park offers wide bike/pedestrian pathways where they can learn to ride.

Ride Log

0.0 Begin at Columbia Valley Elementary School and enter the park via the bike/pedestrian path.

0.09 Right on path to far side of park.

0.38 Left at fork.

0.42 Right to circle far side of park.

0.74 Left to ride the inside circle pathway of the park.

0.84 Right at the fork.

1.05 Right onto main bike/pedestrian path.

1.13 Right to exit park onto SE Sequoia Circle.

1.23 Left onto SE Cardinal Court.

1.35 Enter Wacom Technology and circumnavigate the bike path.

1.74 Left onto SE Sequoia Circle.

1.77 Right onto SE Tech Center Dr.

1.94 Left onto SE Redwood Circle.

2.28 Left at the corner and ride through parking lot at Peet's Coffee.

2.46 Left onto SE Tech Center Dr.

2.81 Right onto SE Sequoia Circle.

2.95 Return to Columbia Valley Elementary School. End ride.

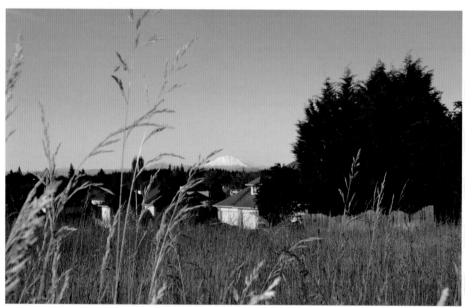

Mount Saint Helens from a high point in Vancouver, WA.

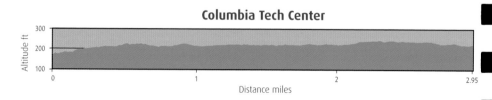

Columbia Tech Center

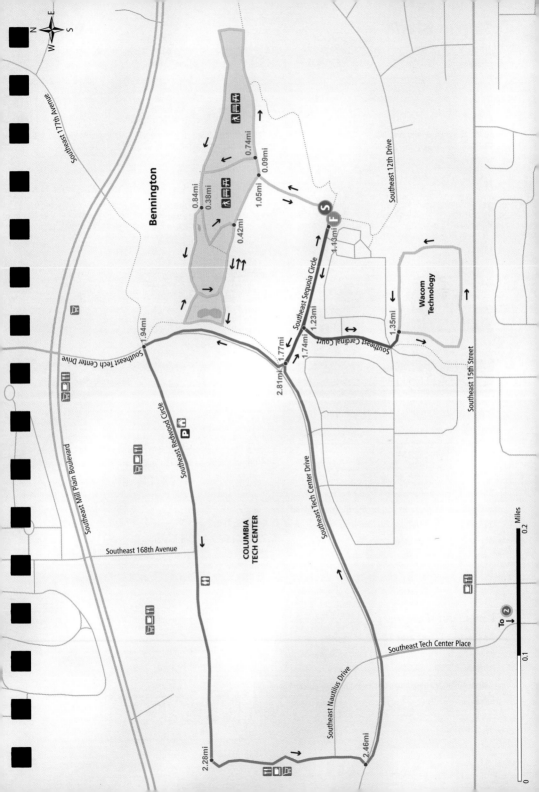

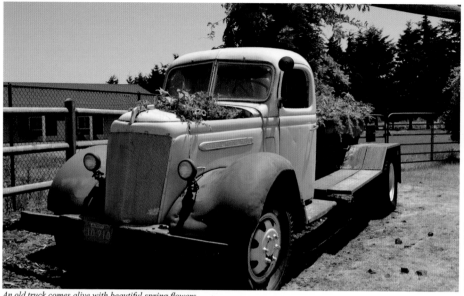

An old truck comes alive with beautiful spring flowers.

At a Glance

Distance 38.2 miles   **Elevation Gain** 365'
Distance from Downtown Portland 13 miles

Terrain

Primarily paved roadways. The roads become rougher in Columbia County on the outer end of the island. At the end of the paved roadways there are dirt roads that can be navigated by mountain bike.

Traffic

Minimal motor vehicles; some farm vehicles.

How to Get There

By car, take US 30 west toward St. Helens. Turn right onto Sauvie Island Road/NW Sauvie Island Bridge. Parking in a lot at the foot of the bridge.

By public transportation, take Bus #17 toward St. Johns.

Food and Drink

There are several places to stop along the route at convenience stores and cafés, but they are a bit of a distance from each other. Be sure to have plenty of water and some snacks with you.

Side Trip

Forest Park, St. Johns neighborhood.

Where to Bike Rating

About...

Sauvie Island is a rural sanctuary just north of downtown Portland. It is a favorite weekend ride of cyclists because of the flat, low-traffic roads. The island is predominantly farmland, and the interior is home to flocks of migrating birds. Beyond the paved roads on the north side of the island are several beaches. Be sure to bring bike repair equipment as there are no bike shops (and no gas stations) on the island.

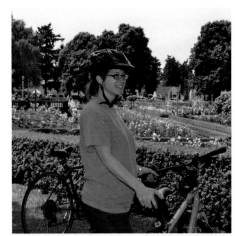

Portland is the City of Roses...they seem to grow everywhere without effort.

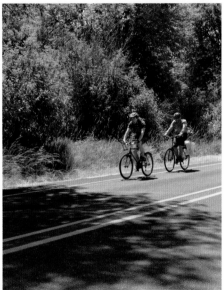

Sauvie Island is a great get-away for day trippers and beach lovers.

This ride will take you on almost all of the paved roads on the island. The route on the northern side of the island takes you along the Columbia River where you'll ride next to the dike. The southern side of the island travels along the Multnomah Channel where you'll ride along the top of the dike and see houseboat communities on one side and farms on the other.

The Sauvie Island Wildlife Area is a bird watcher's paradise. The wetlands are wintering grounds for 1.3 million migrating ducks and geese. About 50 bald eagles find the island to be their idyllic winter nesting spot and can be seen from November to February. If you are lucky, you may see some of the nesting osprey that have built their large nests atop several of the telephone poles. Be sure to take some time to stop and access one of the elevated structures where you can read some history about the island or take a walk to the interior of the island along unpaved pathways.

Fishing, boating, sun-bathing, and cycling bring many people to the island of approximately 2,000 year-round residents. About four miles beyond the end of NW Reeder Road there are beaches, one of which is a popular clothing-optional beach. The most colorful time to ride on the island is in the summer and early fall, but the island has good cycling year-round. The only time I avoid this ride is in mid-winter when the head winds can be quite strong.

There are farms and nurseries, sheep and cattle ranches. Several of the commercial farms allow pick-your-own blueberry and strawberry fields. In the fall, Sauvie Island is a great place for a Sunday ride to pick the perfect pumpkin.

Ride Log

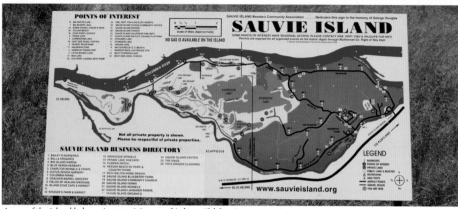

A map of the island helps orientate visitors to this beautiful farming community.

0.0 Begin at the parking lot on the island riding south on N Gillihan Rd.

6.08 Right onto NW Reeder Rd heading along the north side of island.

8.5 Enter Columbia County; the road gets distinctly rougher. The road follows the Columbia River to your right.

10.6 Sauvie Island Eastside Check Station; enter the wildlife area observation area on foot.

11.3 Look up! There is an osprey nest atop the telephone pole that has been a favorite of local bird watchers for years.

12.0 Climb the short hill over the levy and an expansive view of river greets you.

12.3 The paved road ends. Be sure to look out for another osprey nest on a telephone pole where the pavement ends. Turn around and head back along the same road.

18.5 Join up with N Gillihan Rd again. Veer right and follow signs toward Bailey Nursery and Sauvie Island School.

20.6 Oak Island Rd meets NW Reeder Rd; continue straight.

22.9 Right onto Sauvie Island Rd and ride on the southern side of the island down to beaches.

29.6 Pavement ends just beyond the telephone pole. The beaches are beyond this point. Turn around and head back in the same direction.

36.4 Intersection of NW Reeder Rd and Sauvie Island Rd; continue on NW Reeder Rd back to the parking lot on NW Gillihan Rd.

38.2 Return to parking lot. End ride.

> P1 Osprey nests
> P2 Bird watching
> P3 Fruit farms - pick your own berries and pumpkins (seasonal)

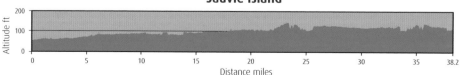

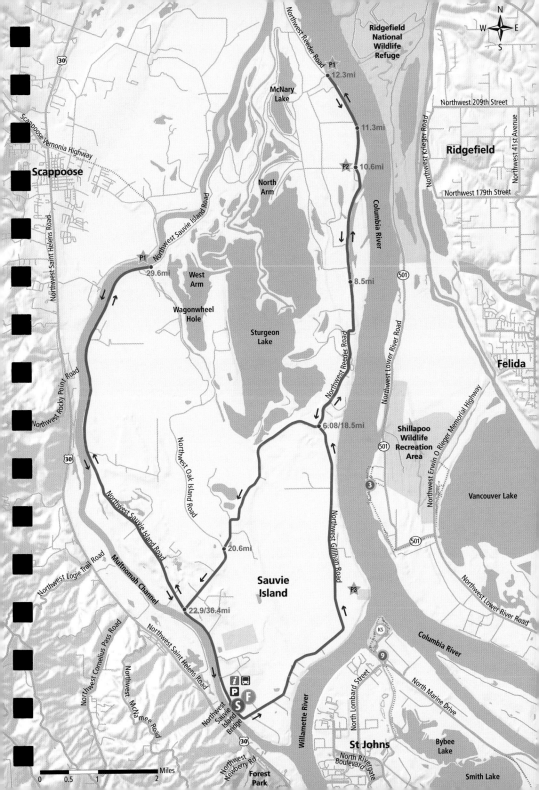

Smith and Bybee Lakes to Kelley Point Park Ride 9

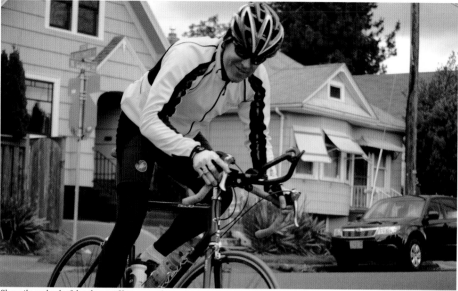

Sly smile and colorful style meet Vancouver Avenue.

Image Matt Wittmer

At a Glance

partially

Distance 27.7 miles   **Elevation Gain** 735′

Distance from Downtown Portland 1.9 miles

Terrain

Smooth, paved streets and paved bike/pedestrian paths some of which will be rough.

Traffic

Moderate urban traffic along most of the streets. The route also accesses bike/pedestrian pathways at the two major parks.

How to Get There

By car, take the Broadway Bridge east, slight right onto N Weidler Street then right onto NE Wheeler Avenue. On-street parking or in the Rose Quarter parking garage.

By public transportation, take TriMet MAX Red, Blue, or Green line to the Rose Quarter Transit Center station.

Food and Drink

There is a small coffee shop at the MAX station and plenty of restaurants at the beginning and end of the ride. There are public restrooms at Smith and Bybee lakes and also at Kelley Point Park.

Side Trip

Visit the University of Portland campus or explore downtown St. Johns.

Links to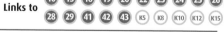

Where to Bike Rating

About...

Not very far from downtown Portland and within easy bicycling distance is the quiet area of Smith and Bybee lakes. A short ride beyond this is beautiful Kelley Point Park at the mouth of the Columbia River. If you like to ride, picnic, sightsee, and hike, this is the perfect ride for you to plan for a warm, summer day. This wonderful nature ride north of Portland has plenty to see and do at the two quiet parks along this route.

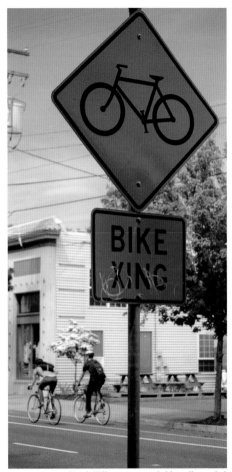

North Williams is remarkably well-traveled.
Image Matt Wittmer

Begin your ride at the Rose Quarter MAX station and ride north toward St. Johns. These urban streets with wide bike lanes are designed for bicycles. N Williams Avenue is a very popular bicycling corridor. You'll also find plenty of bicycling traffic along N Willamette Boulevard. Many of the people who live in this section of town commute by bicycle to school and work.

Just after passing the University of Portland, take a right onto N Portsmouth Avenue and travel through the urban landscape until you come to the Columbia Slough Trail where you will leave traffic behind. Quickly you will find yourself in a quiet park behind the Wastewater Treatment Plant. This trail will bring you to the bike path that parallels the road. Ahead you will see a railroad bridge. Look for the sign indicating that Smith and Bybee lakes are left. Cross the street with care and pass through the concrete barriers onto the unused road. This section of the road is gravelly but most road bikes should be able to handle the terrain. Ride along the railroad tracks. There are numerous hiking trails below the road. At the restrooms you will find bike racks to park your bike if you would like to take a hike down to the lakes.

The path comes up to N. Marine Drive as you exit the lakes area. Here you will encounter very little traffic on weekends as this is the industrial area of the Port of Portland, where cars and containers are unloaded from ships. The bike/pedestrian pathway is very wide and flat. At the end of the pathway, cross onto the street. The access road to Kelley Point Park will be a short ride ahead.

At the far end of the park is the convergence of the Willamette and Columbia rivers and you can see the south end of Sauvie Island. Some people enjoy swimming in the rivers, but the current can be dangerous. There are numerous picnic tables and quiet enclaves in the park. If you are lucky you may see a large ship leaving port for the open waters of the Pacific Ocean.

Ride Log

0.0 Begin at corner of NE Wheeler and NE Multnomah streets and ride north on NE Wheeler St.

0.2 Right onto N Williams Ave bike lane.

2.2 Cross N Killingsworth St through bike-access point to continue on N Williams Ave.

2.5 Left onto NE Ainsworth St.

4.0 Right onto N Willamette Blvd.

4.3 Cross through the bike-access island to turn left onto N Willamette Blvd.

5.9 Right onto N Portsmouth Ave.

7.3 Cross Columbia Blvd; right at bottom of hill onto N Columbia Court to access the Columbia Slough Trail.

7.5 Left onto bike path directly ahead and follow the path around the wastewater treatment plant to the right.

7.9 Right over the bridge to cross Columbia River Slough, then left onto paved portion of the path.

8.3 Right along N Portland Rd; path parallels road.

8.9 Cross N Portland Rd just before railroad bridge.

10.0 Exit lake area; continue straight along path which comes up to N Marine Dr.

12.3 Trail ends; right to cross street and travel on road to Kelley Point Park.

12.7 Enter Kelley Point Park.

13.0 Left at parking lot onto bike/pedestrian path.

14.0 Right fork to ride to the end of the path; reverse direction.

14.2 Right to continue on path.

 P1 University of Portland

14.3 Right onto access road to exit park.

14.7 Left onto N Marine Dr to retrace route back to lake area.

17.0 Continue along bike/pedestrian path through Smith and Bybee lakes.

18.1 Cross N Portland Rd, then right along bike path.

18.7 Left to enter Columbia Slough Trail.

19.0 Right to cross bridge over Columbia Slough.

19.1 Left after bridge to continue along Columbia Slough Trail.

19.6 Exit trail onto N Columbia Court.

19.7 Left onto N Portsmouth up hill to the traffic light and cross Columbia Blvd and take a right onto the sidewalk going in the opposite direction of the traffic; follow the sidewalk to access the Peninsula Crossing Trail.

19.9 Left to access Peninsula Crossing Trail.

20.2 Cross over Fessenden St.

20.7 Cross over Lombard St.

21.0 Path ends at N Carey Blvd. Continue straight.

21.1 Left onto N Willamette Blvd.

23.7 Left on N Ainsworth St.

25.1 Right on N Vancouver Ave.

27.7 Return to the corner of NE Wheeler and NE Multnomah streets. End ride.

Smith and Bybee Lakes to Kelley Point Park

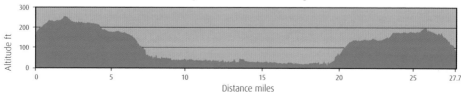

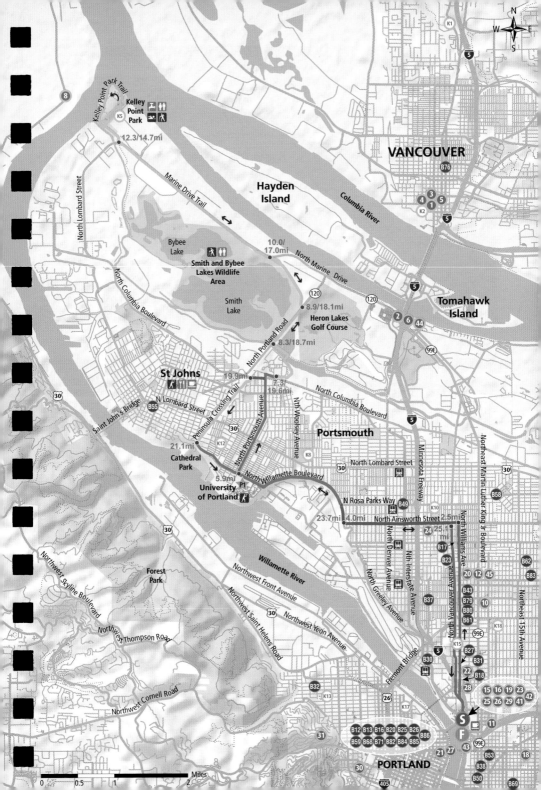

N
W · E
S

VANCOUVER

K1

B76

8

Kelley Point Park Trail
Kelley Point Park
K5
12.3/14.7mi

North Lombard Street

Marine Drive Trail

Hayden Island

Columbia River

K2
4 3 5
1

5

Bybee Lake

North Columbia Boulevard

Smith and Bybee Lakes Wildlife Area

North Marine Drive

10.0/17.0mi

Smith Lake

5

Tomahawk Island

120

120

8.9/18.1mi
Heron Lakes Golf Course

2 6 44

8.3/18.7mi

North Portland Road

99E

30

St Johns

19.9mi

7.3/19.6mi

North Columbia Boulevard

Peninsula Crossing Trail

North Portsmouth Avenue

Nth Woolsey Avenue

Portsmouth

5

N Lombard Street

B55

30

Saint John's Bridge

K12

K8

21.1mi

Cathedral Park

North Lombard Street

B58

30

Minnesota Freeway

5.9mi

North Willamette Boulevard

University of Portland
P1

Northeast Martin Luther King Jr Boulevard

Northeast 15th Avenue

30

N Rosa Parks Way

B49

23.7mi 24.0mi

North Ainsworth Street

2.5mi

K10

24 25.1

30

North Denver Avenue

Nth Interstate Avenue

North Greeley Avenue

B17

B823

North Vancouver Avenue

North Williams Ave

20 12 45

B62

B83

Forest Park

Willamette River

Northwest Front Avenue

B37

B43
B79
B80
B61

10

99E

K18

Northwest Skyline Boulevard

Northwest Saint Helens Road

Northwest Yeon Avenue

30

K15

B27

B31

Northwest Thompson Road

Fremont Bridge

B30

5

B22
28
B818

15 16 19 23
25 26 29 41 42

Northwest Cornell Road

B32

K13

26

K17

21 27

S
F

11

43

99E

B853

18

31

30

PORTLAND

B12 B13 B16 B20 B25 B26 B86
B59 B68 B71 B82 B84 B85

B38

B50

B69

405

Miles
0   0.5   1   2

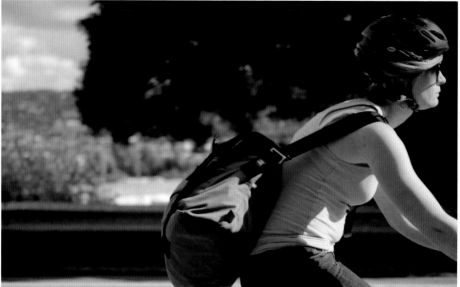

Willamette Boulevard approaches the picture perfect.   Image Matt Wittmer

At a Glance

Distance 15.0 miles   **Elevation Gain** 455'
Distance from Downtown Portland 3 miles

Terrain

Paved streets are smooth with short sections of concrete and cobblestones.

Traffic

Many quiet bike-friendly residential streets and a couple of heavier traveled main roads.

How to Get There

By car, take the Broadway Bridge east; left on NE Grand Avenue (becomes Martin Luther King Boulevard) to NE Failing Street. On-street parking.

By public transportation, take Bus #6 from downtown Portland to the Failing Street bus stop.

Food and Drink

There are several stopping places that provide the opportunity for a bring-your-own picnic or buy-as-you-ride re-fueling at convenience stores, grocery stores, cafés, food carts, and pubs along the route.

Side Trip

Smith and Bybee Wetlands Natural Area, the Columbia Slough, Pier Park, Cathedral Park, Kelley Point Park.

Links to (9) (11) (12) (16) (19) (20) (22) (23) (24) (41) (45) (K7) (K8) (K12) (K14)

Where to Bike Rating

About...

This wonderful ride along Willamette Boulevard, with the working waterfront on one side and quiet residential streets on the other, takes you by parks, the University of Portland campus, and gives you a tour of downtown St. Johns. You'll experience several elements of Portland's bike infrastructure that allow you to ride your bike through busy sections of the city without having to tangle with traffic and cross two busy streets on bike/pedestrian bridges.

St. Johns is located in North Portland on the tip of the peninsula formed by the confluence of the Willamette and the Columbia rivers. St. Johns was originally a separate city that was merged with Portland in 1915. Upon entering St. Johns there is a conspicuously placed sign in the traffic median that reads "Welcome to the Peninsula, Gateway to Nature."

The University of Portland (UP) is a private, Roman Catholic university that was founded in 1901 and today has a student body of about 3,600 students. It is widely known for its soccer program, which won the 2002 and 2005 Division I NCAA Women's Soccer Championships. The campus is located on Waud's Bluff overlooking the Willamette River.

The two major pedestrian walkways that cross over busy I-5 and North Going Street are excellent examples of early bike/pedestrian infrastructure in the city. The North Going Street Bridge has a steep corkscrew curved path that leads up to a narrow bridge. It can be navigated by bicycle, but if others are present, it may be best to walk your bike along this connection.

The North Failing Street Bridge is wider and straighter. However, the bike path ends directly in front of the stairs on the opposite side and riders must

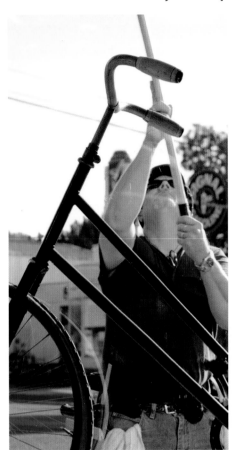

Weir's Cyclery in St. Johns, established in 1925.
Image Matt Wittmer

use caution not to over-shoot the landing. Children and less-experienced cyclists would be wise to walk their bikes across this bridge.

The ride provides wonderful, sweeping views of the city from the campus of the University of Portland and at several other places along the route. There are a couple of parks to stop by and rest or have a picnic. There are food carts along Killingsworth Street, and cafés and an ice cream shop along Mississippi Street. My favorite food cart is PDX671 which offers pacific island fare with a northwest twist. Downtown St. Johns is a great place to lock up your bike and take a stroll around an old fashioned downtown. Many of the signs have been left intact from the 1950s.

Ride Log

P1 Columbia Slough
P2 Failing Street Pedestrian Bridge
P3 N Going Street Pedestrian Bridge
P4 Willamette Bluff
P5 University of Portland
P6 Alberta Arts District

0.0 Begin at NE Failing and MLK Blvd, ride west along NE Failing St.

0.8 Enter the bike ramp for the pedestrian bridge.

0.9 Continue ½ block to the sidewalk between the Kaiser Permanente building and the parking lot.

1.0 Left onto N Montana Ave.

1.05 Right onto N Overlook Blvd up to N Interstate Ave.

1.1 Left onto N Interstate Ave.

1.2 Right onto Fremont and enter Overlook Park.

1.4 Loop the park, exit, and ride the sidewalk in the opposite direction of the traffic along N Interstate.

1.5 Left onto Overlook Blvd.

1.6 Left onto Melrose Dr.

1.8 Left onto N Concord Ave.

2.1 Dogleg left at N Skidmore, descend the hill and cross N Going St via the cork-screw pedestrian bridge. Exit right, and continue on N Concord.

2.6 Left onto N Killingsworth.

3.3 Right onto N Willamette Blvd.

3.9 Left to remain on N Willamette Blvd by riding through the curb cut island.

7.2 Right at N Burlington into downtown St. Johns.

7.22 Right at N Syracuse.

7.26 Left at N Leavitt.

7.3 Right at N Ivanhoe St.

7.32 Left onto N Charleston.

7.4 Left onto N Lombard through town.

7.5 Left onto N Baltimore.

7.55 Left onto N Ivanhoe.

7.6 Cross over N Philadelphia Ave onto N Burlington.

7.6 Left at N Syracuse (to avoid the hill on N Burlington).

7.9 Right onto N Leavitt.

8.0 Left onto N Princeton.

8.05 Right onto N Richmond.

8.1 Left onto N Willamette Blvd.

9.7 Right into the University of Portland campus; left at Buckley Center Auditorium toward the river.

10.2 Return to the school entrance; right onto N Willamette Blvd.

11.6 Right onto N Willamette Blvd (N Rosa Parks continues straight).

12.3 Left onto N Killingsworth.

12.9 Right onto N Concord and cross N Going St via the corkscrew pedestrian bridge; continue along N Concord.

13.6 At the end of N Concord, follow the bike sharrows left onto N Overlook Blvd crossing N Interstate Ave.

14.0 Left onto N Montana.

14.05 Right onto the sidewalk at the end of the parking lot.

14.1 Access the N Failing St pedestrian bridge.

15.0 Remain on N Failing St returning to NE Martin Luther King Blvd. End of ride.

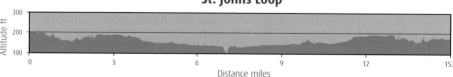

St. Johns Loop

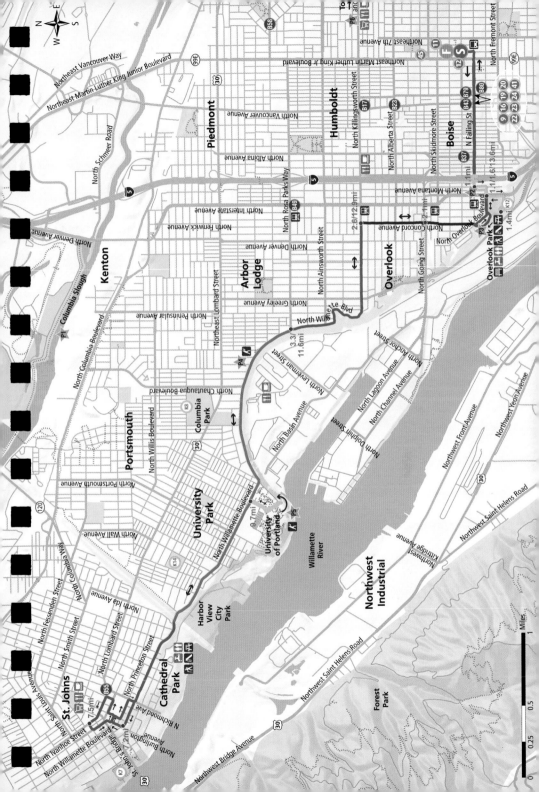

Walls of Pride Art Loop

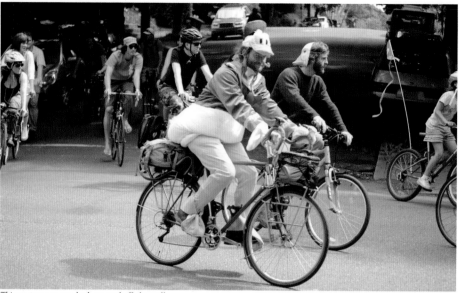

This route oozes art, both on, and off, the wall.

Image Matt Wittmer

At a Glance

Distance 10.7 miles **Elevation Gain** 540'
Distance from Downtown Portland 2.4 miles

Terrain

Smooth paved urban streets many with bike lanes.

Traffic

Low-traffic streets most of the ride with short sections of moderate traffic on wide streets.

How to Get There

By car, take the Broadway Bridge east, continue onto N Weidler Street; turn right onto NE Martin Luther King Boulevard, left onto NE Multnomah Street, right at the third cross street onto NE Seventh Avenue. On-street parking or in one of the parking garages close by.

By public transportation, from downtown Portland take the Blue, Red or Green line east to NE Seventh Avenue TriMet MAX station.

Food and Drink

Plenty of options for food and drinks along the ride route.

Side Trips

Explore the Alberta Arts District or the historic Mississippi District, both teeming with art galleries, restaurants, and small shops.

Links to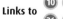

Where to Bike Rating

About...

Portland's buildings have many public murals some of which celebrate the vibrant African-American community and are known as the Walls of Pride. RACC, the Regional Arts and Culture Council, has funded many wall murals in the City. Other murals are community or neighborhood projects designed to provide public art spaces. Street murals are painted on street intersections as strategies to slow traffic in the neighborhood. This short ride with minor elevation is designed to provide riders with ample opportunity to enjoy the art-scape.

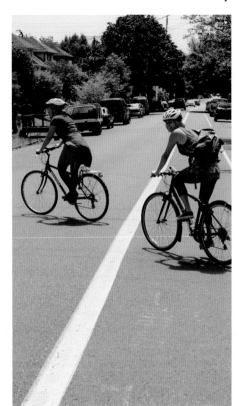

Flat, safe, quiet, NE.   Image Matt Wittmer

Ride south along NE Seventh Avenue, cross I-84 via NE 12th Avenue. Turn from NE Irving Street to NE 24th Avenue where you will find the first murals along NE Everett, Davis, and Flanders streets. This is a very creative section of the city and several of the small shops have taken advantage of blank walls that front onto parking lots to create lively art spaces. This neighborhood is worth a walk-around to visit some of the small shops and restaurants.

The corner of NE Glison Street and NE 24th Avenue has a very colorful building with ample bicycle parking out front and a terrific mural of Cuban culture. Before leaving this area you will encounter one of the street intersection murals with a bright yellow sun pattern.

Travel north through residential neighborhoods to the far end of this route to find an abundance of wall murals in the Alberta Arts District. As you ride, keep an eye open for bicycle art that is exhibited in many of the neighborhood yards.

Along narrow Alberta Street several buildings have murals painted in vibrant colors. The route is designed to keep you off the busiest streets and still bring you past many of the painted murals that grace the sides of build-ings. Of particular note are the murals at the south corner of NE Alberta Street and NE 17th Avenue. Here you will find the Community Cycling Center mural depicting that organization's vision of a healthy, connected community, and the mural of Malcolm X across the street.

At the corner of NE Killingsworth Street and NE Martin Luther King Boulevard you will find another mural that was funded by RACC in the Walls of Pride category. There are several other murals in this general vicinity including some that are inside buildings. If you have an interest in learning of more, they are easy to find with an internet search.

Riding back to the starting point will bring you along popular bicycle traffic corridors and several other wall murals including the one at the corner of NE Seventh Avenue and NE San Raphael Street where there is a wonderful painting that includes bicyclists. Enjoy the scenery!

Ride Log

0.0 Begin at the Seventh Ave TriMet MAX station on the corner of NE Seventh Ave and NE Holladay St; ride south.

0.17 Left onto NE Lloyd Blvd.

0.43 Right onto NE 12th Ave.

0.52 Left onto NE Irving St.

1.1 Right onto NE 24th Ave.

1.3 Left onto NE Flanders St.

1.5 Right onto NE 29th Ave.

1.6 Right onto NE Davis St then right onto NE 28th Ave.

1.7 Left onto NE Everett St.

1.9 Right onto NE 24th Ave.

2.2 Left onto NE Oregon St.

2.3 Right onto NE 22nd Ave then left onto NE Pacific St.

2.4 Right onto NE 21st Ave.

2.9 Right onto NE Hancock St.

3.4 Left onto NE 30th Ave then right onto NE Tillamook St.

3.5 Left onto NE 32nd Ave.

4.2 Left onto NE Klickitat St.

4.9 Right onto NE 17th Ave.

5.5 Jog right at NE Prescott St to remain on NE 17th Ave.

5.6 Right onto NE Going St.

6.2 Left onto NE 29th Ave.

6.4 Left onto NE Alberta St.

6.7 Right onto NE 22nd Ave.

6.8 Left onto NE Sumner St.

7.0 Left onto NE 18th Ave and cross NE Alberta St.

7.1 Right into alley way behind buildings fronting on NE Alberta St then right onto NE 17th Ave.

7.4 Left onto NE Killingsworth St.

8.2 Left onto NE Mallory Ave.

8.6 Left onto NE Going St.

8.8 Right onto NE Sixth Ave.

9.3 Left onto NE Beech St. then right onto NE Seventh Ave.

10.7 Return to corner of NE Seventh Ave and NE Holladay St. End ride.

P1 Alberta Arts District
P2 Mississippi District
P3 NE Everett, Flanders, David Street murals
P4 NE Glison and 24th Avenue Cuban mural
P5 28th and NE Alberta Street murals
P6 17th and NE Alberta Street murals
P7 Killingsworth and MLK Blvd mural
P8 NE Sixth and Failing Street mural
P9 NE Seventh and San Raphael mural

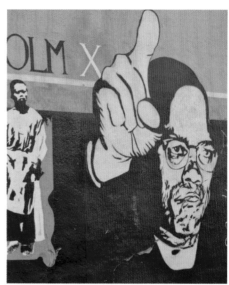

This Malcolm X mural is one of the early public murals in Northeast Portland.

Walls of Pride Art Loop

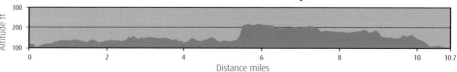

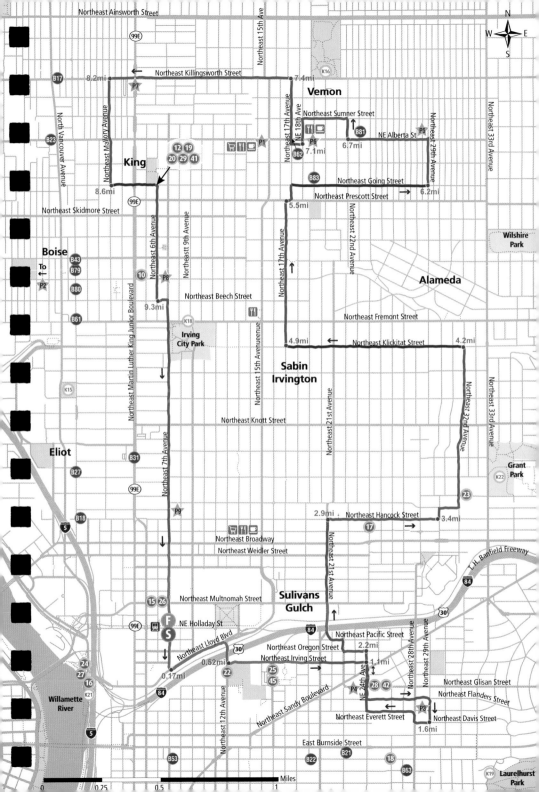

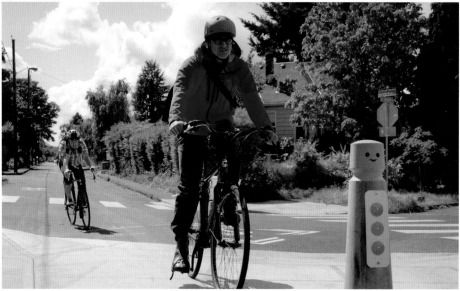

Two cyclists speed past a smiling bollard at Holman Pocket Park.

Image Matt Wittmer

At a Glance

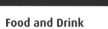

Distance 9.2 miles   **Elevation Gain** 340′

Distance from Downtown Portland 3.3 miles

Terrain

Smooth well-maintained streets. Flat with the highest elevation at 236 feet.

Traffic

Though some of the streets are well-traveled by automobiles, there are plenty of low-traffic streets that meander through the neighborhoods.

How to Get There

By car, take Burnside Street east across the Burnside Bridge then left onto NE Grand Avenue which becomes NE Martin Luther King Boulevard. Right onto NE Going Street. On-street parking.

By public transportation, take Bus #6 along Martin Luther King Boulevard to the intersection of NE Wygant Street. Walk half a block down to NE Going Street.

Food and Drink

Lots of opportunities to fuel up along N Alberta Street, N Killingsworth, 42nd Avenue, and at the intersection of NE Cully Boulevard and NE Prescott Street. There are restrooms and drinking fountains at Fernhill Park. The wonderfully fragrant Delphenia's Bakery is on the corner of NE 42nd Avenue and NE Going Street.

Side Trip

Alberta Arts and historic Mississippi Districts, Woodland Park, Columbia Slough wetlands.

Links to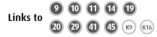

Where to Bike Rating

About...

Located in the Northeast quadrant of the city this ride passes by several parks and through lovely Northeast Portland neighborhoods. You will ride on NE Going Street, one of the popular neighborhood greenways also known as bike boulevards, and onto a cycle track, which separates cyclists from the motor vehicles via a raised track. You can also access this ride via several bus routes.

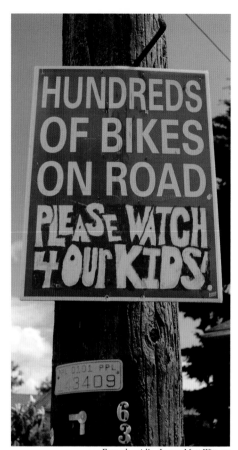

Enough said!   Image Matt Wittmer

Begin by taking the #6 Bus disembarking on NE Martin Luther King Boulevard at NE Going Street. Proceed east along NE Going Street. This route brings you by several urban green spaces.

The first park you will come to is Woodlawn Park which is bisected by a wooden bridge and has paved pathways, several shaded park benches, picnic areas, and a playground. The second park is Alberta Park located along NE Ainsworth Boulevard where the roadway is separated by a landscaped mall. This is the location of a weekly Bike Polo game every Sunday afternoon at 3pm and often on Wednesday evenings. The official city-sanctioned play space is the tennis courts allowing the players to engage in this rough and tumble game on a smooth surface and fenced off from the rest of the park . Players converge on the park, polo mallets in hand, ready to rumble. After some contentiousness, the city and players worked out an agreement to allow players to bring "adult beverages" to the park as long as they are in covered containers.

Fernhill Park is the third park along the route and marks the approximate mid-point of the ride. This large park has tennis courts, a big playground with a popular tire swing, and varying topography that the

cyclist can ride by and admire while remaining on the relatively flat road surface. This park is a popular location for high school cross-country track meets because of its hills and dips. There is also a well-favored designated dog park on the far side next to the softball field.

On the return trip along NE Going Street two schools have large fields and playgrounds. King School Playground is not a designated park, but is used as such by the neighborhood because of its large field. King School is also the site of the annual Good in the Hood event and the kick-off parade of Pedalpalooza each June. Another popular playground is located at Rigler Elementary School, and though it is small, the neighborhood children enjoy the play structures here.

Ride Log

0.0 Begin at NE Going St and MLK Blvd, ride east on NE Going St.

0.7 Left onto NE 17th Ave to the corner of NE Alberta St.

0.9 Cross NE Alberta St and dog leg left at NE Killingsworth St to remain on NE 17th Ave.

1.5 Dog leg left at NE Holman St to remain on NE 17th Ave.

1.7 Left onto NE Junior St.

1.9 Right onto NE 13th Ave. Cross NE Dekum St, then an immediate right onto NE Claremont Ave around the Woodland Park Condos and into Woodland Park.

2.1 Left onto NE Oneonta St.

2.3 Left to cross NE Dekum St to continue on NE Durham St. NE Durham St ends at NE Holman St where tiny Holman City Park is located.

2.6 Left around the park and then right onto N 13th Ave.

2.7 Left onto NE Ainsworth St. NE Ainsworth St ends at NE 37th Ave at the entrance to Fernhill Park.

4.0 Left onto NE 37th Ave.

4.1 Right onto NE Holman St at roundabout keeping Fernhill Park on your right.

4.3 At 41st Ave you will find another roundabout. Take a right continuing with the park on your right hand side.

4.5 Follow the road as it turns into NE Simpson Ct after crossing NE 42nd Ave.

4.7 Left onto NE Simpson St.

5.5 Right at NE 60th Ave and cross NE Killingsworth St.

6.1 Right onto NE Going St.

6.4 Right onto NE 55th Ave at the Rigler School playground.

6.5 Left onto NE Wygant St.

6.6 Left onto NE 52nd Ave. Basically you will have gone around the playground.

6.7 Right onto NE Going St again.

6.9 Dogleg left at NE 47th Ave to remain on NE Going St. Cross busy NE 42nd Ave and remain on NE Going St.

7.7 Left at NE 33rd Ave via the cycle track and jog right onto NE Going St.

9.1 Pass by King Middle School playground.

9.2 Return to NE Martin Luther King Blvd and NE Going St. End of ride.

 P1 Alberta Arts District
P2 Mississippi District
P3 King Elementary School

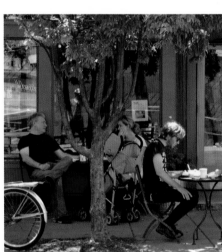

A sidewalk café on NE Alberta Street is a wonderful way to spend an afternoon.

Fernhill Park

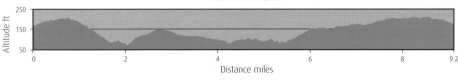

Altitude ft

Distance miles

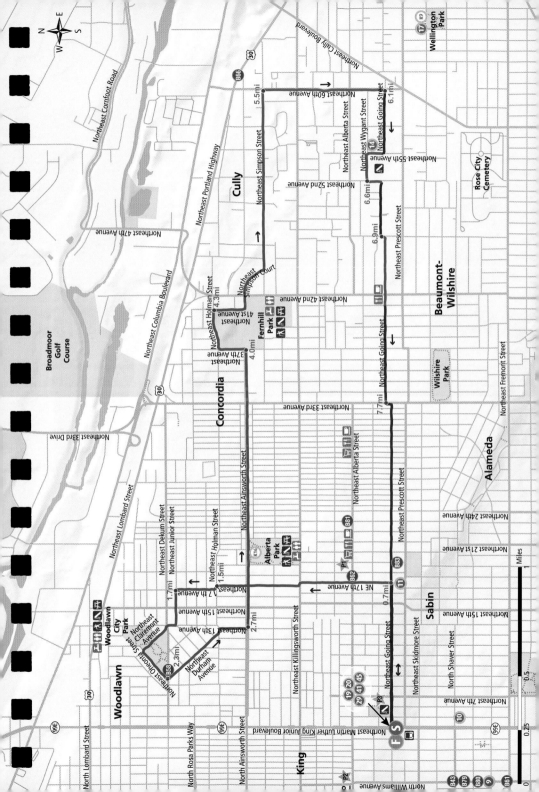

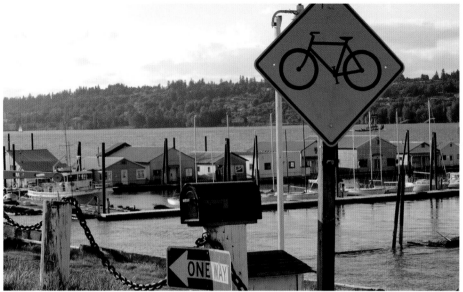

It doesn't get much better than idyllic Marine Drive.

Image Matt Wittmer

At a Glance

Distance 15.4 miles   **Elevation Gain** 280′
Distance from Downtown Portland 12.7 miles

Terrain

Smooth, well-maintained streets.

Traffic

Low-traffic streets with bike lanes and bike paths.

How to Get There

By car, Morrison Bridge east then I-5 N/I-84 E/US-30 E ramp to I-84 to The Dalles; exit 8 to merge onto I-205 N toward Portland airport; exit 24A for Airport Way W toward Portland airport; merge onto NE Airport Way; slight right to stay on NE Airport Way. Parking available at Aloft Hotel and at the shopping center.

   By public transportation, take the TriMet MAX Red line toward airport to Cascade station.

Food and Drink

There are restrooms and drinking fountains at Blue Lake Regional Park.

Side Trips

Visit Blue Lake Regional Park; ride the full length of Marine Drive; stop and watch the planes take off and land.

Links to

Where to Bike Rating

About...

This flat course highlights the efforts to keep Portland's water clean. Ride Marine Drive along the magnificent Columbia River; visit beautiful Blue Lake Regional Park, and return to Cascade station with views of the Columbia Slough. Much of this ride travels the wide lanes through industrial parks that have low traffic on weekends. The rest of the ride is along bike paths with bike and pedestrian traffic, but no motor vehicles.

Beginning at Cascade station this ride will bring you through the commercial/industrial section of northeast Portland which offers terrific roads to ride on weekends when vehicular traffic is almost nonexistent. Along the way you will have views of Mount Hood from several vista points. If you choose a clear day to ride, the mountain peak appears to rise out of the Columbia River along Marine Drive.

Visiting somewhat remote sections, you will have views of the Johnson Lake Property and the Columbia Slough, both of which are great places to do some bird watching. Blue Lake Regional Park is the perfect point to stop for a picnic and enjoy the lake. There are plenty of picnic tables available at the park, or just rest beside the shore and enjoy the view. Leaving the park, ride along the bike path to the far side and exit through the chain link fence onto NE Interlachen Lane. The return trip brings you along Marine Drive near the airport. It is quite a sight to have a plane land while you are riding on the switchback leaving the bike path. The airport is ahead of you and the planes come in directly overhead. You may want to stop for a while just to experience the thrill.

Return to Cascade station via NE Airport Way

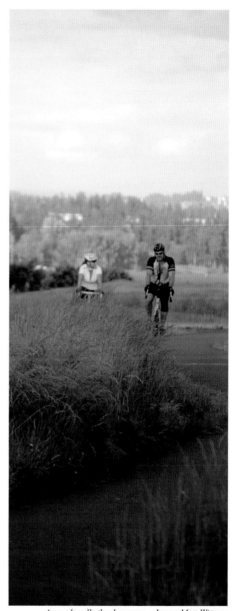

A couple rolls the day away.   Image Matt Wittmer

which has a wide bike lane. If you didn't plan a picnic at Blue Lake Regional Park, there are plenty of restaurants and courtyards at Cascade station to spend some time relaxing.

Ride Log

P1 Columbia Slough
P2 Portland International Airport

0.0 Begin at Cascade MAX station.

0.1 Cross the TriMet tracks; right onto NE Mount St. Helens Ave.

0.4 Left onto NE Alderwood Rd.

0.6 Left onto NE Glass Plant Rd; reverse direction.

1.0 Cross NE Alderwood Rd to Johnson Lake Property; reverse direction.

1.5 Right onto NE Alderwood Rd.

1.6 Left onto NE 105th Ave.

2.2 Right onto NE Airport Way.

4.3 Left onto NE 152nd Pl.

4.4 Right at cul-de-sac onto bike path.

4.6 Cross NE 158th Ave onto NE Cameron Blvd.

5.1 Right onto NE 166th Ave.

5.2 Cross NE Airport Way to Columbia Slough; reverse direction; right onto NE Airport Way.

6.0 Left onto NE River Side Parkway.

6.4 Left onto NE 185th Ave.

6.7 Right onto NE Marine Dr bike path.

7.8 Right onto NE Blue Lake Rd.

8.0 Enter park.

9.0 Right onto NE Interlachen Lane to exit park.

9.2 Left onto NE Marine Dr bike path.

12.1 Cross NE Marine Dr via bike/pedestrian traffic signal.

12.8 Cross NE Marine Dr at NE 122nd Ave to access bike path on opposite side.

14.4 Via switchback cross NE Marine Dr to bike path on opposite side.

14.8 Right at roundabout onto NE Lombard St which becomes NE Mt. Hood Ave.

15.1 Left onto NE Cascade Parkway.

15.4 Return to starting point. End ride.

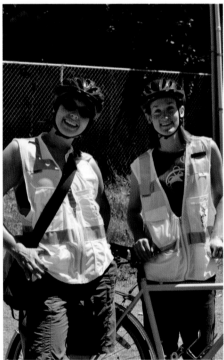

The Ground Water Tour ride leaders enjoy a few moments rest along the side of the road.

Ground Water Well Tour

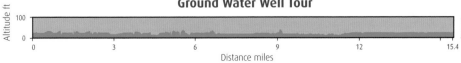

Altitude ft

Distance miles

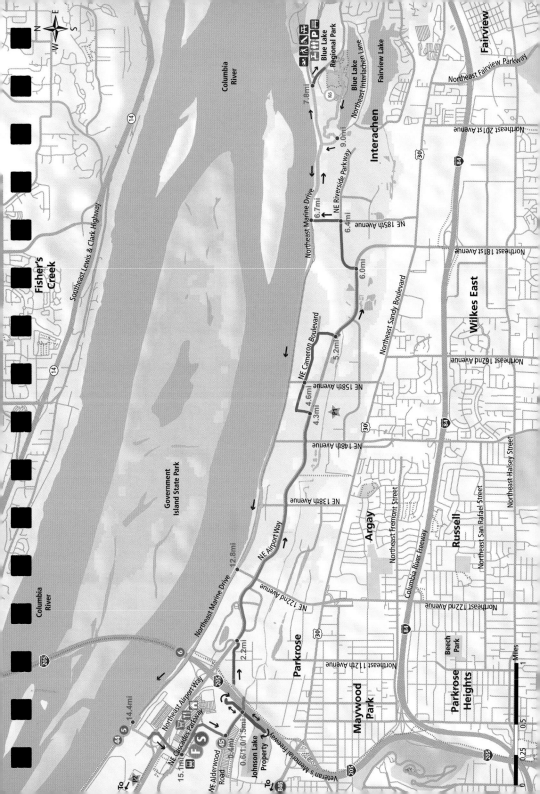

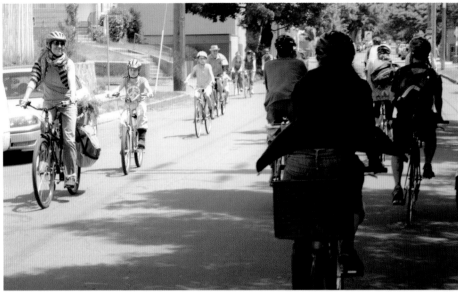

Just another weekend afternoon in Portland.

Image Matt Wittmer

At a Glance

Distance 6.9 miles   **Elevation Gain** 385'
Distance from Downtown Portland 6.0 miles

Terrain

Paved streets, mostly flat.

Traffic

The traffic in this neighborhood can be quite busy on the arterial roadways of Cully Boulevard and Fremont Street, but the residential areas have mostly local traffic that travels slowly.

How to Get There

By car, take the Burnside Bridge east, left onto NE Grand Avenue which becomes NE Martin Luther King Boulevard after a slight turn; right onto NE Fremont Street, left onto NE 42nd Avenue, right onto NE Prescott Street, and the third left will be NE 55th Avenue. On-street parking.

By public transportation, take Bus #75 to Killingsworth and 52nd; walk south on 52nd to Prescott Street.

Food and Drink

There are restrooms and drinking fountains at Wilshire Park. Numerous opportunities for snacks, drinks, and ice cream can be found on Cully Boulevard and Fremont Street.

Side Trip

Be sure to spend some time in the parks and playgrounds along the route.

Links to

Where to Bike Rating

 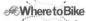

About...

Three schools with playgrounds, several churches, and one cemetery dot this urban figure eight. Though some of the roads are a little narrow, there are plenty of opportunities to enjoy quiet neighborhoods along low-traffic streets. The route has several doglegs which are very common in Portland's urban streetscape and add interest to the ride. Some of the roads are designated bike-friendly and are marked with sharrows.

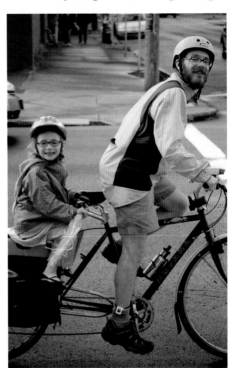

Father and daughter on the move.   Image Matt Wittmer

Cully Neighborhood

The Cully neighborhood parks include Sacajawea Park, Rigler Community Garden, and Whitaker Ponds Natural Area. Cully has a smaller amount of parkland per capita than the rest of Portland, but it has several school playgrounds that are used often by neighborhood residents. The Rose City Cemetery is located in the southwest corner of the neighborhood and contains the Japanese Cemetery. Rigler Community Garden provides a community gathering place where both children and adults can garden.

Rigler School

Named for Frank Rigler, a professor who became superintendent of schools in Portland, this school has a very diverse student body. With a large Hispanic population the school offers a two-way Spanish immersion program. The playground that surrounds the school is a popular place for neighborhood children to gather and play.

Harvey School Elementary School

The school was named for Harvey Whitfield Scott who became editor of The Oregonian newspaper in 1865,

the same year he passed the bar exam. He was a pioneer and a historian in addition to being a newspaper editor. He was also the brother to Abigail Scott Duniway, a famous suffragette. Mount Scott, an extinct volcano in Happy Valley was named for him, and a statue of Harvey Scott stands at the top of Mount Tabor, another extinct volcano.

Joseph Meek Technical School

This alternative high school offers vocational and academic programs in a small classroom environment. The school is named for Joseph Meek, a trapper, law enforcement officer, and politician who traveled to Oregon in 1840. He was acclaimed as a storyteller and intrepid adventurer during his lifetime and was one of the first to take a wagon train up the Oregon Trail to the Willamette Valley. Joseph Meek witnessed the transformation of the West from a wilderness to organized territory.

Ride Log

0.0 Start at Rigler Elementary School on NE 55th Ave, there is parking available on the street.

0.4 Left onto NE Alberta at Word of Life Community Church; follow the bike sharrows on NE Alberta St.

.045 Right onto NE 52nd Ave.

0.5 Right onto NE Emerson St.

0.6 Left onto NE 53rd Ave.

0.7 Right onto NE Killingworth St. This is a busy street with a wide bike lane. Pass the Trinity Church and School on the left.

1.0 Right onto NE 60th Ave. This is a narrow road with no bike lane, but cars travel slow.

1.5 Follow NE 60th to the intersection of NE Cully Blvd and NE Prescott St. This intersection has a grocery store, pharmacy, convenience store and other retail stores. Continue through the intersection onto Cully Blvd.

2.4 Left onto NE Fremont at the traffic light. This is a busy intersection; do a box turn if necessary.

2.8 Left onto NE 71st Ave and go past the Calvary Presbyterian Church.

3.3 Continue to Prescott and take a left.

3.5 Pass Harvey Scott Elementary School (has a great playground) and Northeast Baptist Church across from the school.

3.7 Cross over NE Cully Blvd at the traffic light where NE Prescott St and NE Cully Blvd meet.

4.1 Right onto NE 55th Ave and return to Rigler School.

4.4 Continue down NE 55th Ave.

4.6 Left onto NE Alberta St.

4.65 Dogleg left on NE 52nd to remain on NE Alberta St.

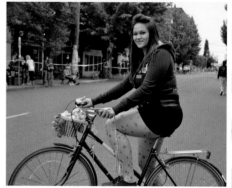
Pedalpalooza brings out the joy of cycling.

 P1 Rose City Cemetery, Japanese Cemetary
P2 Rigler Elementary School
P3 Harvey Scott Elementary School
P4 Joseph Meek Technical School

4.8 Dogleg left on 47th to remain on NE Alberta St.

5.0 Dogleg left at NE 42nd Ave to remain on NE Alberta St. Joseph Meek Technical High School is on the right.

5.4 Left onto NE 35th Ave.

5.7 Left onto NE Skidmore St at Wilshire Park.

6.1 Cross over NE 42nd Ave.

6.5 At NE 49th Ave make a dogleg left to stay on Skidmore.

6.6 Another dogleg turn at NE 52ndAve to stay on Skidmore.

6.8 Left onto NE 54th Ave. Rigler School is directly across the street from NE 54th.

6.9 Right onto NE Prescott St.

6.9 Immediate left onto NE 55thAve. End ride.

Cully Neighborhood Figure Eight

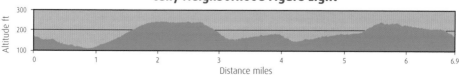

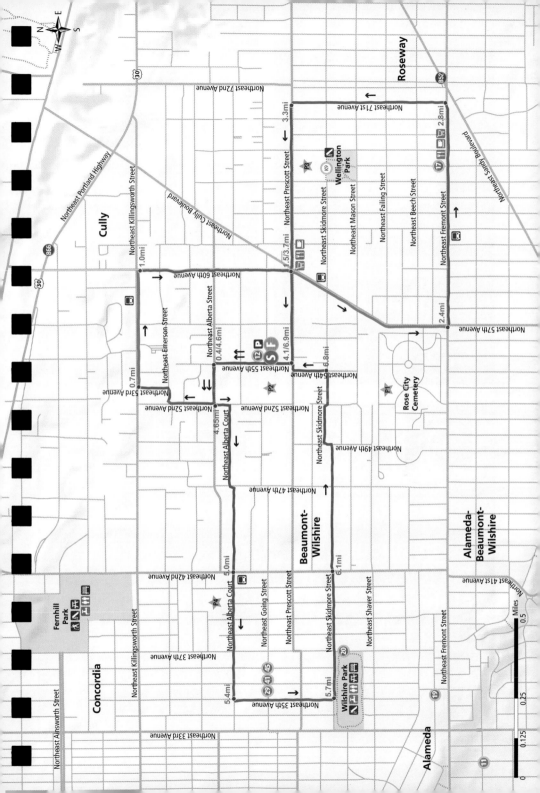

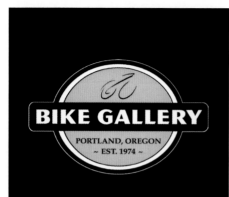
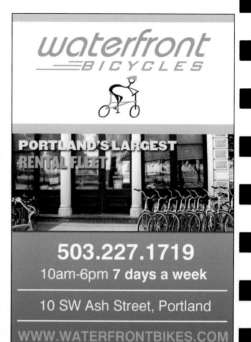
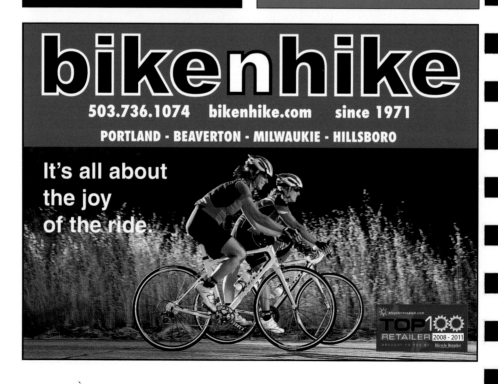

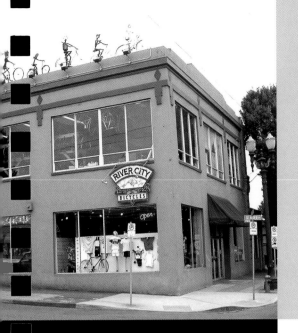

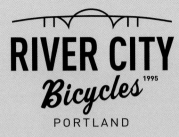

RIVER CITY *Bicycles* 1995

PORTLAND

ORIGINAL
706 SE MLK BLVD
503.233-5973

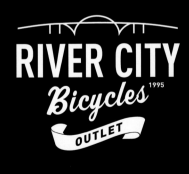

RIVER CITY *Bicycles* 1995
OUTLET

OUTLET
534 SE BELMONT ST
503.446.2205

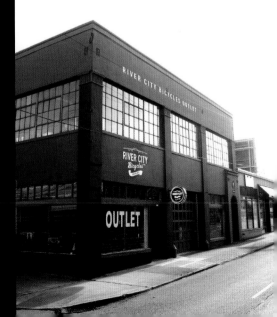

BICYCLE TRANSPORTATION ALLIANCE

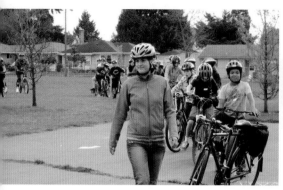
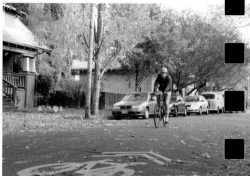

PORTLAND IS THE #1 CITY FOR BIKING IN AMERICA.

More people are bicycling in Portland than ever before, and the demand for safe, healthy streets is loud and clear. With hundreds of miles of bike paths, neighborhood greenways, cycletracks, and trails connecting all parts of the city, Portland is a great place to ride a bike, whether you're a seasoned commuter, weekend cruiser, or brand new rider.

The Bicycle Transportation Alliance makes your ride better every day.

As Portland's leading bike advocacy organization since 1991, the BTA has fought for safer streets, better bike infrastructure, and stronger laws to protect people who ride. Our mission is simple: to transform communities through bicycling by making the ride safe, convenient, and accessible.

BTA MEMBERS POWER THE BIKE MOVEMENT.

We advocate for a world-class bike network. We teach kids to be safe, confident, legal riders. We encourage more people to ride bikes.

BTA members make it all possible.

Help make Portland a better place to ride a bike for you and thousands of new riders every year by becoming a member of the Bicycle Transportation Alliance today.

MEMBERSHIP BENEFITS!

Year-round discounts at 80+ bike shops and other businesses • Members-only ride discounts • Exclusive invites to special events • And more!

btaoregon.org/join

• • • • • • • • • • • • MORE • • • • • • • • • • • • •
btaoregon.org/memberbenefits

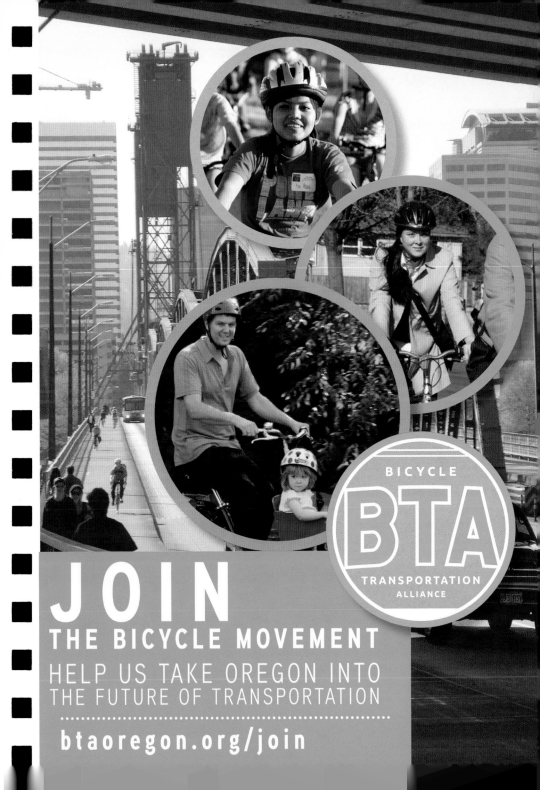

JOIN
THE BICYCLE MOVEMENT
HELP US TAKE OREGON INTO
THE FUTURE OF TRANSPORTATION

btaoregon.org/join

BICYCLE
BTA
TRANSPORTATION
ALLIANCE

Downtown & Theme Rides

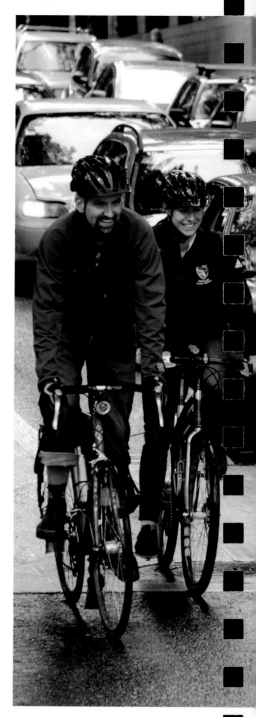

Downtown Portland has a myriad of opportunities for adventurous souls and the rides in this section provide a thematic exploration of the area. Interested in art? Museums? Food carts? Or are you a secret fan of The Simpsons television show? All can be found in this section and are designed for you to ride again and again as you explore many of the stops along the way on both sides of the Willamette River that bisects Portland.

Some of the most popular bicycling paths run along the edge of the Willamette River and cross several of the bridges that connect the east and west sides of Portland. Most popular with cyclists are the Steel and the Hawthorne bridges. The Willamette Bike Trail on the west side, the East Esplanade, and the Springwater Corridor have all been known to have traffic jams of pedestrians, bicyclists, runners, and skaters on warm summer weekends. Patience is highly recommended when traveling these sections during busy periods. They are critical bicycle arteries in Portland, however, and allow for ease of access to many of the treasures that Portland offers.

Portland is a city that is very easy to navigate by bicycle. Downtown streets have bike lanes, traffic moves slowly, and vehicles all negotiate their place on the street with relative ease. Along with abundant bike parking, Portland is a great city to explore by bicycle stopping along the way to lock up and visit whichever café, museum, or food cart you choose.

Getting to and from Portland is also important, and this section contains a very practical route to the airport from downtown Portland. So if you are planning a visit to Portland, you can begin and end your bicycle adventure at the airport.

Come explore the Platinum Bicycle City of Portland and acquaint yourself with (or explore anew) all of the treasures it has to offer by traveling around town on your bicycle sampling the craft beer, delicious food, amazing art, and beautiful parks.

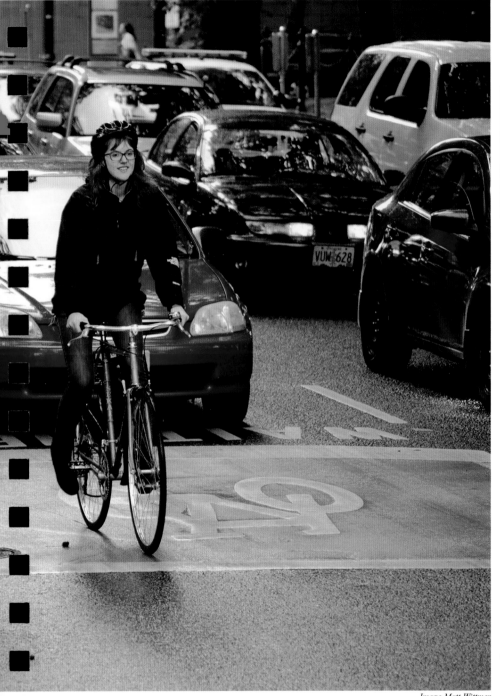

Image Matt Wittmer

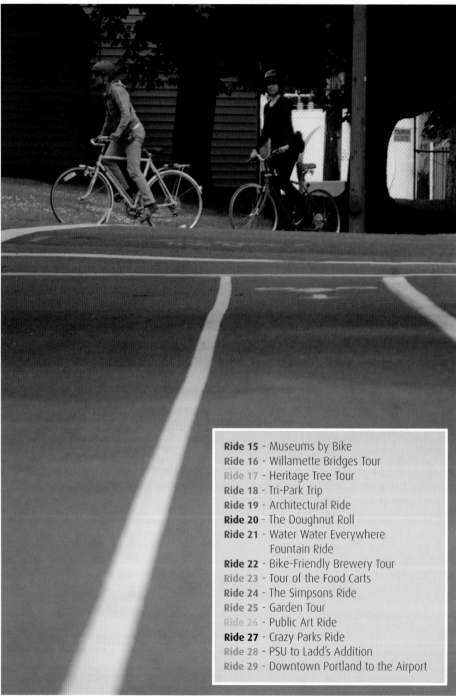

Ride 15 - Museums by Bike
Ride 16 - Willamette Bridges Tour
Ride 17 - Heritage Tree Tour
Ride 18 - Tri-Park Trip
Ride 19 - Architectural Ride
Ride 20 - The Doughnut Roll
Ride 21 - Water Water Everywhere
        Fountain Ride
Ride 22 - Bike-Friendly Brewery Tour
Ride 23 - Tour of the Food Carts
Ride 24 - The Simpsons Ride
Ride 25 - Garden Tour
Ride 26 - Public Art Ride
Ride 27 - Crazy Parks Ride
Ride 28 - PSU to Ladd's Addition
Ride 29 - Downtown Portland to the Airport

Image Matt Wittmer

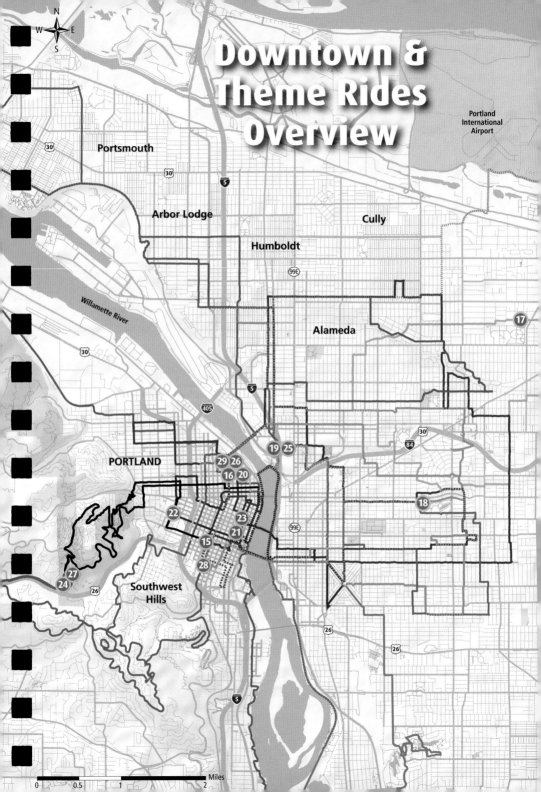

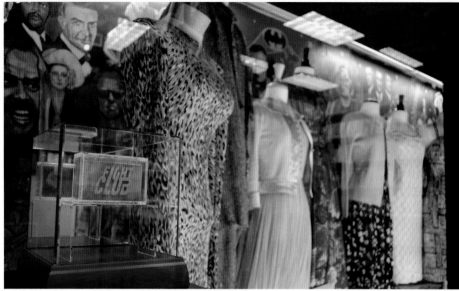

Mike's Movie Memorabilia has all sorts of cool stuff for movie buffs.

Image Matt Wittmer

At a Glance

Distance 10.6 miles   **Elevation Gain** 622′

Distance from Downtown Portland 0.4 miles

Terrain

Smooth paved urban streets, many with bike lanes or sufficiently wide enough to accommodate all types of traffic.

Traffic

Urban streets with moderate traffic.

How to Get There

By car, park in any of the downtown Portland garages. This ride begins six short blocks from the heart of downtown Portland.

By public transportation, from downtown Portland take the green line south to SW Jefferson Street and walk/ride three blocks southwest.

Food and Drink

Plenty of options for food and drinks along the route. There is a fabulous farmers market on the campus of Portland State University every Saturday just two blocks south of the starting point.

Side Trips

Visit the Architectural Center, the Stark Vacuum Museum, and the Toy Museum all located on SE Grand Avenue (which is not bike-friendly – but all are worth a visit).

Links to 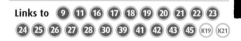 9 11 16 17 18 19 20 21 22 23 24 25 26 27 28 30 39 41 42 43 45 K19 K21

Where to Bike Rating

About...

There are wonderful museums in Portland, some traditional and some quirky. This ride will help you to navigate the downtown streets of the city and bring you to interesting and unique museums along the way. Any of the museums along this route are worth a visit, though to do them all justice you may have to make this trip more than once.

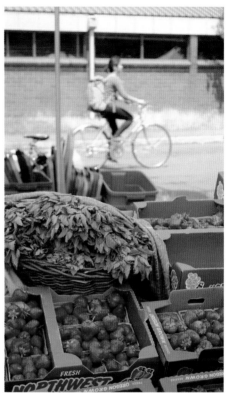

No city pairs bicycles and farmer's markets better than Portland. Image Matt Wittmer

The ride starts at the Oregon Historical Museum where there are permanent exhibits of the Lewis and Clark Expedition and is one block south of the Portland Art Museum. You'll ride down SW Park Avenue along the South Park Blocks. This area is very popular with pedestrians and cuts a green corridor through downtown Portland.

When you turn onto NW Couch Street you'll find two quirky museums: The Church of Elvis and the Ground Control Arcade. The Church of Elvis is built into the side of a building and is barely the size of a doorway. Across the street a short distance is the Ground Control Arcade that boasts vintage arcade games. When riding the streets downtown you will be traveling slowly, often no faster than the automobiles. It is perfectly acceptable to "take the lane" and ride among the cars.

Couch Street will bring you to the waterfront and the Oregon Maritime Museum. Cross the Steel Bridge via the bike/pedestrian ramp to the east side of the city and ride through the Lloyd District on your way to Belmont Street where you'll find Mike's Movie Memorabilia. The glass cases are filled with old movie posters and memorabilia, just like the sign promises. You can

also rent a movie while you visit. The ride over to Belmont Street will take you along neighborhood streets designed for ease of bicycling through the city.

Your return trip is through Ladd's Addition, a beautiful section of the city with gardens and roundabouts. Here you will find the Hat Museum on SE Ladd Avenue which you can visit by appointment and take a trip through history via hundreds of vintage hats. The streets of Ladd's Addition are wide and tree-lined. On an autumn day the sun shines through the bright yellow foliage making your bike ride all the more wonderful.

Crossing over the Hawthorne Bridge you come through downtown Portland once again past the Wells Fargo Building where there is a permanent exhibit of the Pony Express days. You'll return to the starting point of the ride where you can spend some time at the farmers market.

Ride Log

P1 PSU Farmer's Market
P2 Portland Art Museum
P3 Oregon Historical Museum
P4 Pioneer Courthouse Square
P5 North Park Blocks
P6 Ground Control Arcade
P7 Church of Elvis
P8 Oregon Maritime Museum
P9 Mike's Movie Memorabilia
P10 The Hat Museum
P11 Toy Museum
P12 Stark Vacuum Museum
P13 Wells Fargo Bank

0.0 Begin at the corner of SW Park St and SW Jefferson St. Ride down South Park Blocks.

0.6 Cross W Burnside St and continue straight onto NW Park St (North Park Blocks). Right onto NW Couch St.

1.0 Right onto NW Naito Parkway.

1.3 Left at NW Pine St to cross NW Naito Parkway. Left onto Waterfront Park Bike Path.

1.8 Right over Steel Bridge bike/pedestrian path.

1.9 Slight left at end of bridge to ride up bike path switchbacks.

2.1 Left at top of path onto sidewalk. Left at bike signal traffic light onto NE Lloyd Blvd (cross diagonally).

2.3 Right onto NE Wheeler St and ride through Rose Garden TriMet Transit Center. Follow green bike lanes.

2.4 Right onto NE Multnomah St.

2.7 Right onto NE Seventh Ave.

3.0 Left onto NE Lloyd Blvd.

3.3 Right onto NE 12th Ave to cross highway.

3.4 Left onto NE Irving St.

3.6 Right onto NE 16th Ave. Cross NE Sandy Blvd and E Burnside St.

4.0 Left onto SE Ankeny St.

4.9 Left onto SE 32nd Ave. Cross E Burnside St.

5.0 Right onto NE Couch St.

5.5 Right onto NE 41st Ave. Cross E Burnside St to continue on SE 41st Ave.

5.9 Jog right at SE Stark St to remain on SE 41st Ave.

6.0 Left onto SE Morrison St.

6.1 Right onto SE 42nd Ave.

6.2 Left onto SE Yamhill St.

6.3 Left onto SE 44th Ave.

6.4 Left onto SE Belmont St.

6.5 Left onto SE 42nd Ave.

6.6 Right onto SE Taylor St.

7.0 Left onto SE 35th Ave.

7.1 Right onto SE Salmon St.

8.1 Left onto SE 16th Ave.

8.3 Jog left at SE Hawthorne Blvd to remain on SE 16th Ave.

8.4 Remaining on SE 16th Ave, right at Ladd's Addition Square Garden then left keeping garden on the left; exit the Square Garden by taking a right on SE 16th Ave.

8.5 Right at Ladd's Addition Circle Garden one block onto SE Ladd Ave.

8.8 Cross SE Hawthorne Blvd onto SE 12th Ave.

8.9 Left onto SE Madison St.

9.6 Cross Hawthorne Bridge onto SW Main St.

10.0 Left onto SW Third Ave.

10.2 Right onto SW Jefferson St.

10.5 Left onto Park St and return to corner of Park and Columbia streets.

10.6 End ride.

Museums by Bike

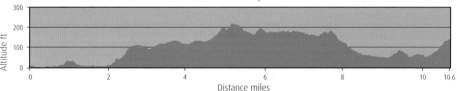

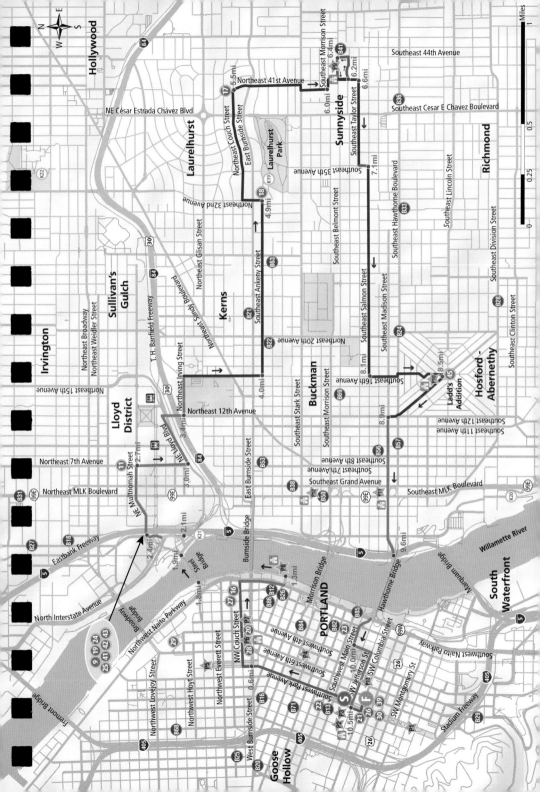

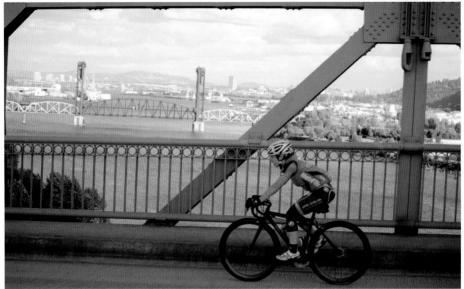

A view south down the Willamette as seen from the St. John's Bridge.   Image Matt Wittmer

At a Glance

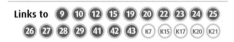

Distance 26.6 miles   **Elevation Gain** 1078′
Distance from Downtown Portland 0.0 miles

Terrain
Smooth, well-maintained street and paths.

Traffic
Low-traffic streets and bike paths.

How to Get There
By car, from Pioneer Courthouse Square in downtown Portland, travel east on SW Sixth Avenue. This road will put you directly in front of Union Station where the ride begins. On-street parking.

By public transportation, take the TriMet MAX Green line toward Clackamas Town Center to the corner of NW Sixth Avenue and NW Hoyt Street. Easily accessible by foot from Pioneer Courthouse Square by walking down SW Sixth Avenue (becomes NW Sixth Avenue after crossing Burnside Street).

Food and Drink
There are restrooms and drinking fountains at Union Station, the East Esplanade near the Hawthorne Bridge, along Waterfront Park, and again at Willamette Park.

Side Trips
Ride the OHSU tram up Marquam Hill; ride the full length of the Springwater Corridor; visit Saturday Market, the University of Portland, and the downtown areas – quaint downtown St. Johns, colorful Sellwood Center, and Portland City Center.

Links to 9 10 12 15 19 20 22 23 24 25 26 27 28 29 41 42 43 K7 K15 K17 K20 K21

Where to Bike Rating

About...

Portland is a city of bridges with 10 crossing the Willamette River. Each provides beautiful vistas of the city and points beyond. This ride will bring you over the two most distant bridges – the St. Johns and the Sellwood bridges. Along the way plan to enjoy several parks, popular bike paths, and see the waterfront from both sides of the river.

Beginning at renovated Union Station, travel along NW Naito Parkway where Saturday Market is in full swing on weekends. The traffic will be light as you ride the bike lane to Tom McCall Waterfront Park. Plan to encounter pedicabs, children splashing in the fountain, and lots of waterfront visitors. Along the south-side bike path there are many interesting storefronts. Ride under the Oregon Health and Science University tram that travels up Marquam Hill.

There are a couple of tricky turns on the south side – one where the bike path ends at a parking lot and one after leaving Willamette Park. Look for the Willamette Greenway Trail signs and you can't go wrong. When in doubt, follow the signs to Sellwood. Just beyond the park, ride along the sidewalk in the opposite direction of traffic.

At the end of this narrow section, you will take the lower road half-way down the hill to access the narrow and steep switchbacks that bring you to the Sellwood Bridge. Ride or walk your bike on the sidewalk. There is a sign indicating that bikes are in the roadway, but most people ride or walk on the sidewalk. The view of Portland from the Sellwood Bridge is magnificent.

After crossing the bridge, ride back toward Portland via Springwater Corridor along the east side of the river to the Steel Bridge. Here you will leave the river for a while to ride north to St. Johns where you'll cross the

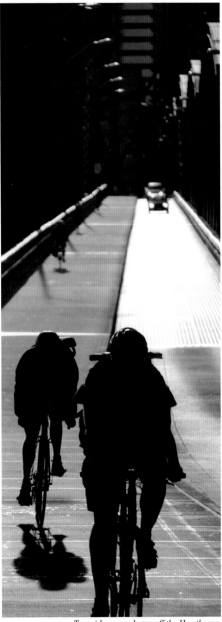

Two riders race home off the Hawthorne.
Image Matt Wittmer

most elegant bridge in Portland – the St. Johns Bridge – and have another sweeping view of the city. Return to Portland through the northwest quadrant of the city.

Downtown & Theme Rides

Ride Log

0.0 Left out of Union Station onto SW Fifth Ave toward downtown Portland.

0.2 Left onto NW Everett St.

0.5 Right onto NW Naito Parkway along waterfront.

1.2 Left at SW Salmon St into Waterfront Park.

1.6 Right onto SW Harbor Way cul-de-sac.

1.7 Left onto SW Montgomery St; at circle continue to river via sidewalk.

2.1 At dead-end, retrace steps short distance; left onto path.

2.2 Right at SW River Parkway, then left onto SW Moody Ave.

3.2 Continue straight onto path at The Willamette Shore Trolley Bancroft St station.

3.4 Bike path ends; left along narrow sidewalk to riverfront; right on bike path.

4.6 Enter Willamette Park.

5.1 Exit park via SW Miles Pl.

5.3 Right at end of path, cross tracks up to road.

5.4 Left on sidewalk toward Sellwood.

5.6 Take lower road; half way down access trail to cross bridge. Use sidewalk in opposite direction to traffic.

6.0 Left onto SE Grand; left onto SE Spokane St; immediate right onto Springwater Corridor.

9.1 Springwater Corridor bike path ends; straight along SE Fourth Ave.

9.2 Left onto SE Caruthers St to access Eastbank Esplanade at cul de sac.

11.0 Right before Steel Bridge up switchbacks; left along the sidewalk to traffic light; cross diagonally onto NE Lloyd Blvd.

11.3 Right onto NE Wheeler Ave following green bike lanes.

11.5 Right onto NE Williams Ave.

13.0 Left onto NE Skidmore St.

13.9 Right onto N Concord St to access corkscrew bike/pedestrian crossway, and right upon exit to continue on N Concord.

14.5 Left onto N Killingworth St.

15.1 Right onto N Willamette Blvd; left through bike access to continue on N Willamette Blvd along bluff.

19.0 Right onto N Philadelphia St to cross St. Johns Bridge via sidewalk.

19.8 Left onto NW Bridge Ave.

20.2 Continue straight onto St. Helens Rd.

24.1 Right onto NW Ward Way St.

24.2 Left on NW Vaughn St.

24.7 Right onto NW 24th Ave.

24.9 Left onto NW Raleigh St.

25.4 Right onto NW 19th Ave.

25.5 Left onto NW Overton St.

26.0 Right onto NW Ninth Ave.

26.3 Left onto NW Hoyt St.

26.5 Left onto NW Sixth Ave.

26.6 Return to Union Station. End ride.

 P1 Willamette Park

Please note: Bike shops are not shown on this map as the scale is too large for locations to be discernable. Please see other rides in this chapter for bike shop locations.

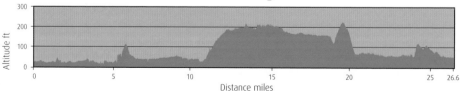

Willamette Bridges Tour

Altitude ft / Distance miles

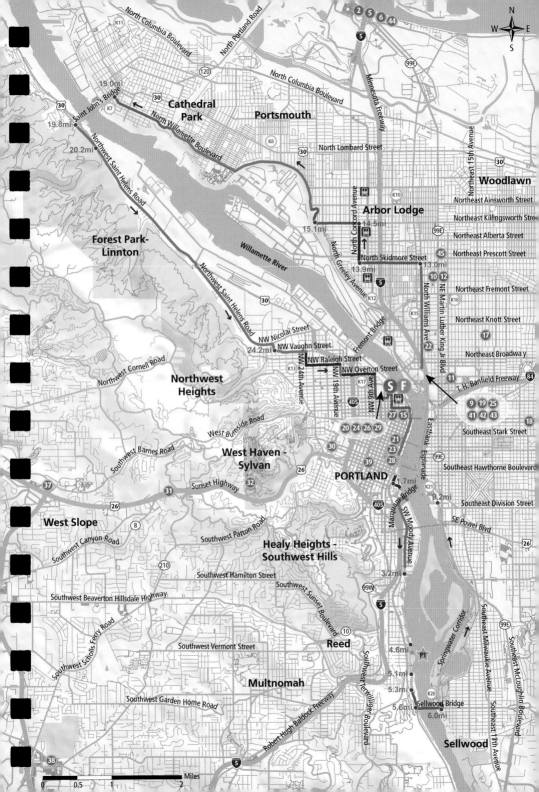

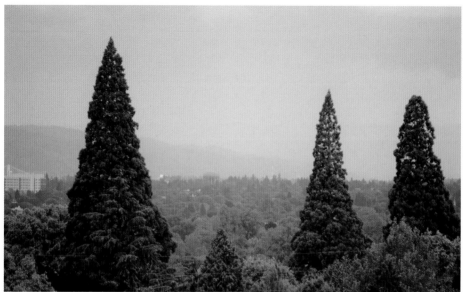

Three city sentinels.

Image Matt Wittmer

At a Glance

Distance 9.2 miles   **Elevation Gain** 262′
Distance from Downtown Portland 7.3 miles

Terrain

Smooth, well-maintained streets.

Traffic

Low-traffic streets with most intersections having crossing lights.

How to Get There

By car, take the Morrison Bridge, left on SE Grand Avenue, right on NE Fremont Street, left onto NE 66th. On-street parking.

By public transportation, take Bus #12 toward Gresham Transit Center to NE Sandy and 67th Avenue (stop #5118) and walk to NE 67th Avenue.

Food and Drink

There are restrooms and drinking fountains at Wellington Park. Though there are many opportunities for food and drinks only short distances from this route, there are none on the route you will travel to visit the noted Heritage Trees.

Side Trip

Like trees? Consider visiting the Children's Arboretum at 10040 NE Sixth Avenue or the Hoyt Arboretum in Washington Park.

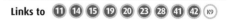

Links to (11) (14) (15) (19) (20) (23) (28) (41) (42) (K9)

Where to Bike Rating

About...

The ride begins at Wellington Park where you'll find a wonderful shaded start to your journey. You will meander through history as you visit some of the oldest, rarest, and most unusual trees in Portland located in picturesque neighborhoods. Most of the Heritage Trees are located on private property and bear a plaque that identifies them by name. To learn more about Heritage Trees in Portland, visit the Urban Forest section of the Parks and Recreation web site at **www.portlandonline.com**.

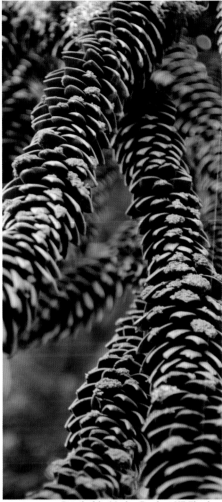

Detail of the Monkey Puzzle at NE Flanders.
Image Matt Wittmer

The tallest tree on the ride is the Carolina Poplar which you will find on NE Couch Street just after crossing NE 41st Avenue. This tree stands at an incredible height of 135 feet and has a circumference of over 19 feet. Another noteworthy tree for its 100 feet of height is the Tulip tree located on NE 24th Avenue.

The most unusual specimen is the Monkey Puzzle tree which you will find on NE Flanders Street just after crossing NE Laurelhurst Place. This Chilean Pine tree has spiny, bizarre branches that overlap and create a mass of branches that would seem impossible to climb. The cones produced by this tree are quite large and can resemble coconuts. This example of the Monkey Puzzle tree stands at 75 feet tall and is over eight feet in circumference.

My favorite tree by far is the European Beech that you will find on the corner of NE Knott Street and NE 18th Avenue. This tree stands at 80 feet and has a girth of over 20 feet. Besides being an incredibly large tree taking over almost the entire front yard, the house that sits behind the tree is one of the most stunning old Victorians in the city.

There are many other noteworthy trees on this ride. Other beautiful trees you'll see include the Weeping Cherry at NE Klickitat Street, the Japanese Red Pine at NE Couch Street and the Hedge Maple on NE Multnomah Street. You may find one of them to be your favorite as you wind your way through these quiet neighborhood streets.

In addition to taking the time to visit all the trees on this route, you'll be riding very close by several parks including Normandale Park, Rose City Park, and Frazer Park all of which offer ample opportunity to stop and enjoy a picnic during your neighborhood tour.

Downtown & Theme Rides

Ride Log

0.0 Begin at Wellington Park and ride east along NE 67th Ave.

0.4 Right on NE Klickatat St.

0.6 Left onto NE 62nd Ave.

0.9 Left on NE Stanton St, then right on NE 63rd Ave.

1.1 Left onto NE Brazee St, then right onto NE Sacramento St.

1.5 Left onto NE 57th Ave, then right onto NE Thompson St.

1.7 Left onto NE 53rd Ave.

2.7 Right onto NE Everett St.

3.0 Left onto NE 47th Ave, then right onto NE Davis St.

3.3 Left onto NE 41st Ave.

3.4 Right onto NE Couch St.

3.6 Right onto NE Laurelhurst Pl.

3.7 Left onto NE Flanders St.

4.0 Right onto NE 32nd Ave.

4.2 Left onto NE Oregon St.

4.5 Right onto NE 28th Ave.

4.7 Left at NE Wasco St and ride through the barriers onto the cul de sac.

4.8 Left onto NE 27th Ave, then right onto NE Multnomah St.

5.0 Right onto NE 24th Ave; at Broadway, ride through the traffic island as indicated for bicycles.

5.4 Left onto NE Tillamook St around the roundabout.

5.7 Right onto NE 18th Ave.

6.3 Right onto NE Klickatat St.

6.5 Left onto NE 21st Ave.

6.6 Right onto NE Regents Dr.

7.2 Right onto NE Shaver St.

8.3 Left onto NE 49th Ave, gravel road for ½ block then right onto NE Mason St.

9.2 Return to Wellington Park. End ride.

P1 Columbia Children's Arboretum
P2 Hoyt's Arboretum
P3 Wellington Park
P4 Carolina Poplar - NE Couch St
P5 Monkey Puzzle - NE Flanders
P6 Tulip Tree - NE 24th Ave
P7 European Beech - Knott and 18th

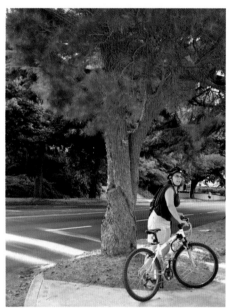

This sharp-eyed rider found the Japanese Red Pine.

Heritage Tree Tour

Altitude ft / Distance miles

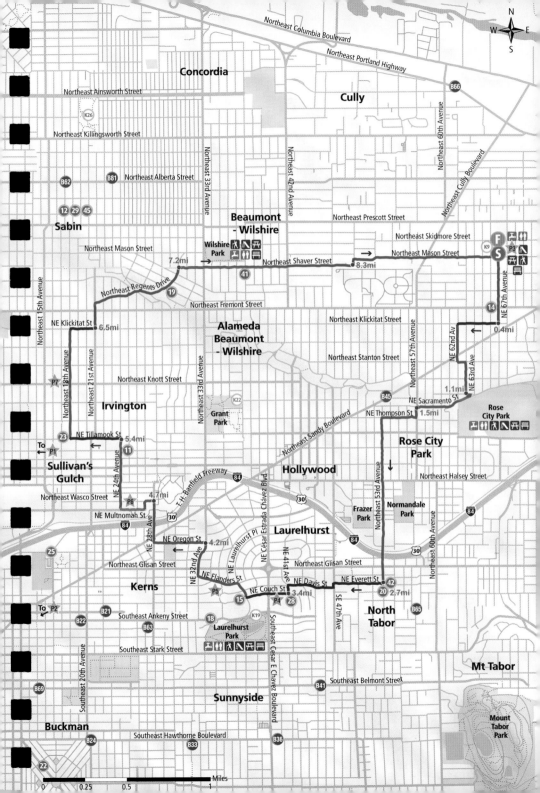

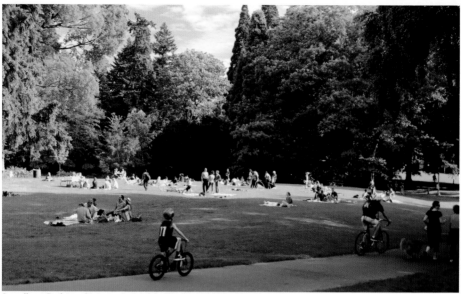

Laurelhurst Park is a shining example of the City Beautiful Movement.

Image Matt Wittmer

At a Glance

Distance 6.2 miles   **Elevation Gain** 260′

Distance from Downtown Portland 3.2 miles

Terrain

Smooth, well-maintained streets with sharrows and bike lanes.

Traffic

Low-traffic streets.

How to Get There

By car, take the Morrison Bridge east; first left onto SE Grand Avenue; right onto SE Stark Street; left onto SE 37th Avenue. On-street parking.

By public transportation, take Bus #15 to SE Belmont Street and SE 37th Avenue, stop #425.

Food and Drink

There are restrooms and drinking fountains at Laurelhurst and Colonial Summers parks.

Side Trip

Oaks Amusement Park, Hawthorne and Belmont Districts, downtown Sellwood, Crystal Springs Rhododendron Garden.

Links to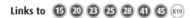

Where to Bike Rating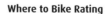

About...

The neighborhoods on the east side of the city have been upgraded to provide bike-friendly infrastructure and encourage low-traffic streets. Many of the streets have way-finding signs for cyclists, sharrows painted on the streets, and traffic signals for easy crossing of busy intersections. Beginning at Laurelhurst Park, one of the largest and most popular parks in Portland, this route will take you along many of the streets that provide safe travel for cyclists.

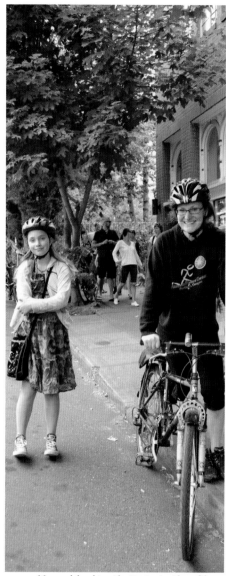

Mum and daughter ride city streets with confidence.

Laurelhurst Park is a great place to being this journey. The park is 31 acres of year-round fun. It includes a pond, a basketball court, a dog off-leash area, horseshoe pit, picnic sites, a playground, a soccer field, tennis courts, and a volleyball court. The large grassy fields are very popular places on warm Sunday afternoons for family picnics, and the pathways are filled with children and adults riding their bikes.

From Laurelhurst Park, begin the loop around southeast Portland and come to Colonel Summer City Park at SE 17th Avenue and SE Taylor Street. This six acre park tucked into the residential neighborhood has similar features to Laurelhurst Park but not as much expanse. Visit the southwest corner of the park to find a large rock from Kelly Butte with a bas relief of Colonel Summers, the commanding officer of the Second Oregon Volunteers Regiment in the Spanish-American War, and the legislator who introduced the bill which later created the Oregon National Guard.

Continue along your ride to Sewallcrest Park at SE 31st Avenue and SE Market Street. Also a small park in a residential neighborhood, this park is a good choice to stop for a snack, to let your dog run in the off-leash section, and enjoy lying back on the grass for a few moments before continuing your journey.

End your ride by taking a spin around Laurelhurst Park where you can enjoy the large shade trees, and the abundance of rhododendrons growing along the pathways.

Ride Log

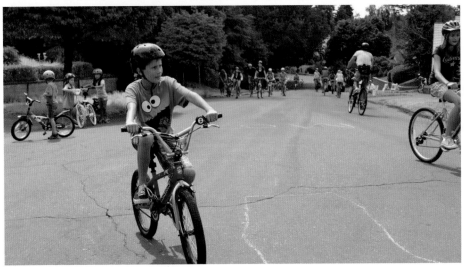

The hill out of Laurelhurst Park is challenging.

0.0 From Laurelhurst Park at SE 37th Ave and Oak St ride west toward SE 33rd Ave.

0.3 Right onto SE 33rd Ave.

0.4 Left onto SE Ankeny St.

1.4 Left onto SE 16th Ave.

1.9 Left onto SE Taylor St.

2.1 Right onto SE 21st Ave then left onto SE Salmon St.

2.8 Right onto SE 32nd Place.

3.3 Right onto SE Grant St then left onto SE 32nd Ave.

3.6 Left onto SE Clinton St.

4.5 Left onto SE 47th Ave; jog at SE Division to remain on SE 47th Ave.

4.9 Left onto SE Harrison St.

5.0 Right onto SE 45th Ave.

5.6 Left onto SE Washington St.

5.7 Right onto SE 43rd Ave.

5.8 Right onto SE Stark St then immediate left onto SE 44th Ave.

5.9 Left onto SE Oak St. Difficult crossing at SE Cesar Chavez Blvd.

6.2 Return to Laurelhurst Park. End ride.

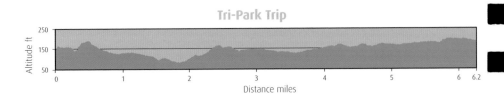

Tri-Park Trip

Altitude ft

Distance miles

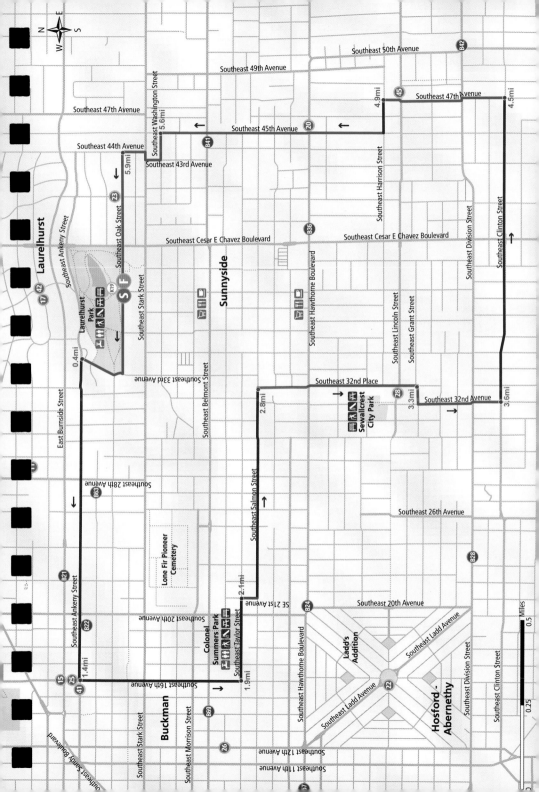

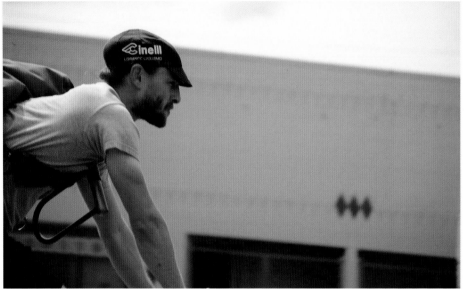

This route rewards a well-trained eye.   Image Matt Wittmer

At a Glance

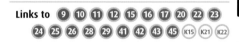

Distance 9.1 miles   **Elevation Gain** 535'
Distance from Downtown Portland 1.9 miles

Terrain
Smooth, well-maintained streets and paths.

Traffic
Low-traffic streets and bike paths.

How to Get There
By car, from downtown Portland take the Steel Bridge east, turn right onto NE Oregon Street, left into NE First Avenue, left onto Multnomah Street, left onto NE Wheeler Avenue. Parking available in the Rose Quarter Parking Garage or on-street.

By public transportation, take any Red, Blue, or Green MAX train east to the Rose Quarter TriMet Transit Center MAX station.

Food and Drink
There are many choices for food and drink along the route. Public restrooms can be found at the Pioneer Place Food Court on SW Fifth Avenue and at both Grant and Irving parks.

Side Trips
Interesting buildings of architectural interest include the Armory in downtown Portland, the Alphabet Historic District near Pearl, and the Skidmore/Old Town Historic District near the waterfront.

Links to 9 10 11 12 15 16 17 20 22 23 24 25 26 28 29 41 42 43 45 K15 K21 K22

Where to Bike Rating

About...

Portland has beautiful neighborhoods of interesting homes. The Grant Park neighborhood is full of large homes with manicured lawns and gardens located on wide and winding streets. Houses on the south side of the ride have views of the city. Alameda is a street that runs generally east/west along a 100 foot ridge in the northeast quadrant of Portland where you will find some of the most stately homes in the City.

Beginning in the Rose Quarter and riding north along NE Williams Avenue, you will be travelling along one of Portland's most popular bicycle commuting corridors. Many residents of the northeast quadrant commute to work and do their grocery shopping exclusively by bicycle. Along Williams Avenue you will also see many examples of bicycle art. Turn right onto NE Going Street and continue your trip along a popular Neighborhood Greenway – a low-traffic residential street designed as a preferred bicycle route. The houses along these corridors are small and quaint.

Turn at NE 22nd Avenue and pick up NE Alameda Street and the neighborhood changes. These houses are large and many were built pre-World War II with the earliest having been built in the mid-1800s. These streets are the Alameda/Irvington/Wilshire neighborhoods.

The wide streets in these neighborhoods are the perfect choice for a sunny Sunday afternoon ride. The mature trees help to shade the wide thoroughfares that amble past neatly landscaped front yards. Ride at a leisurely pace in order to enjoy the unique architecture of the neighborhood.

On the return to downtown Portland, you'll ride

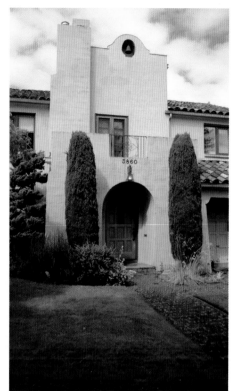

Spanish-inflected architecture on Alameda Street.
Image Matt Wittmer

through Grant Park – the perfect place for a picnic under large shade trees. One unique feature of this park is the fountain on NE 33rd Avenue that has three of the beloved Beverly Cleary characters sculptured in bronze – Ramona, Henry, and Ribsy, the dog. The beautiful sculptures are favorites of children and adults alike.

Once you turn onto NE Seventh Avenue the neighborhood houses begin to get smaller as you travel toward the City Center. You'll ride past Irving Park, another great location for a picnic on top of the small hill dotted with old growth majestic trees. On an autumn day, the grass is blanketed with stunning yellow leaves.

Crossing NE Martin Luther King Boulevard to remain on NE Knott Street brings you through the Boise Elliott neighborhood onto NE Vancouver Avenue, another of the well-travelled bicycle commuting corridors and returns you to the Rose Quarter starting point.

Ride Log

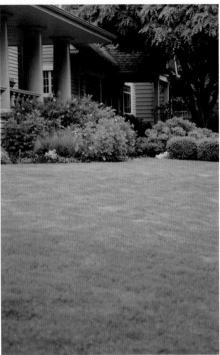

One of dozens of today's perfectly manicured lawns.
Image Matt Wittmer

0.0 Begin at the Rose Garden TriMet MAX station and ride north on NE Wheeler St.

0.16 Slight right onto NE Williams St.

1.79 Right onto NE Going St.

2.04 Cross NE Martin Luther King Jr Blvd to remain on NE Going St.

2.95 Right onto NE 22nd Ave.

3.25 Left onto NE Alameda St. Remain on Alameda. This road curves several times.

4.92 Right onto NE Wiberg Ln.

5.12 Right onto NE Brazee St.

5.87 Cross NE 36th Ave into Grant Park.

6.17 Exit the park in the middle of the block at NE 33rd Ave and cross onto NE Thompson St.

7.53 Right onto NE Seventh Ave.

7.74 Left onto NE Knott St.

7.88 Jog left at NE Martin Luther King Blvd to remain on NE Knott St.

8.21 Left onto NE Vancouver Ave.

8.76 Road becomes NE Wheeler St. Continue to follow back to Rose Garden TriMet MAX station.

9.1 End ride.

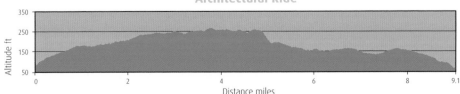

Architectural Ride

Altitude ft / Distance miles

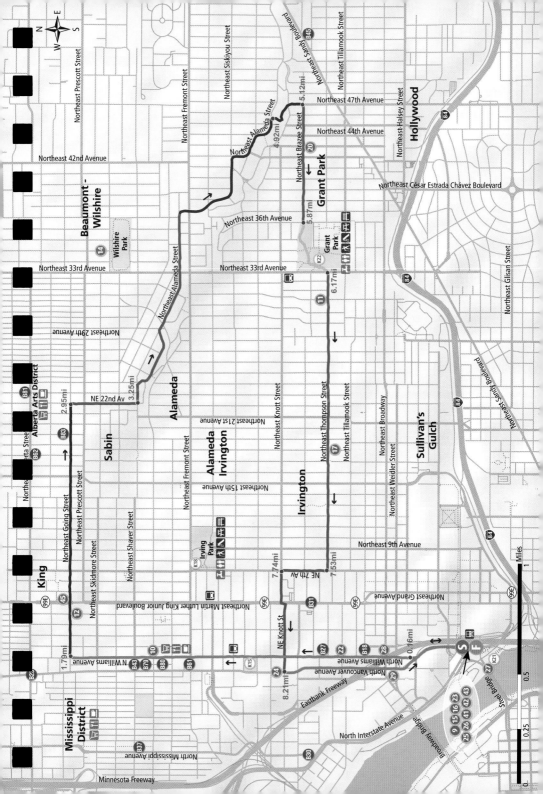

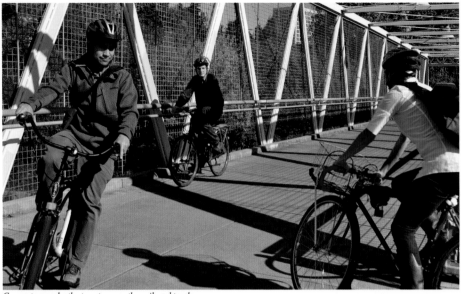

Commuters make the turn to cross the railroad tracks.

At a Glance

Distance 17.7 miles   **Elevation Gain** 850'
Distance from Downtown Portland 0.9 miles

Terrain

Smooth, well-maintained streets, some with train tracks.

Traffic

Low to moderate traffic streets through urban neighborhoods.

How to Get There

By car, from downtown Portland drive north on SW Sixth Avenue and the train station will be directly ahead. On-street parking.

By public transportation, take the TriMet MAX Yellow line train; disembark at NW Sixth Avenue and NW Hoyt Street.

Food and Drink

This ride is all about finding great bakeries, so there are many choices for food and drink along the route. Public restrooms can be found at the Union Station.

Side Trips

Alberta Arts District, Mississippi Historic District, downtown St. Johns, the Belmont District, and the Pearl District are all close by and worth your time to explore.

Links to 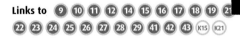 9 10 11 12 14 15 16 17 18 19 21 22 23 24 25 26 27 28 29 41 42 43 K15 K21

Where to Bike Rating

About...

They say that Portland is a town of foodies and this ride highlights the terrific choices for baked goods throughout the city. Ride through all four quadrants to find one bakery in each, but along the way you'll find many more that you will want to visit on a return trip. You may even want to make this loop twice to work off the calories you'll be eating along the way!

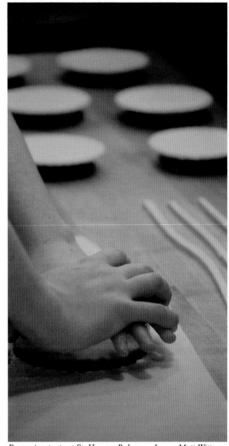

Preparing tarts at St. Honore Bakery.   Image Matt Wittmer

Union Station is a great place to begin. It offers restrooms and a small restaurant in case you need fuel to carry you to the first stop – Voodoo Doughnuts on the corner of SW Third Avenue and SW Ankeny Street. This world famous doughnut shop is a legend in Portland with unique doughnuts such as bacon, maple, and, of course, Voodoo Doll doughnuts. While the shop will do custom orders, they do not ship, so it is not uncommon to see people at the airport with a hot pink Voodoo Doughnut box.

After wiping the powdered sugar from your lips, cross the Willamette River via the Hawthorne Bridge to the southeast quadrant. Hawthorne Boulevard has a bike lane for part of the way, but as you enter the Hawthorne District, the bike lane goes away. Ride beside the cars on this somewhat narrow street. Once past the downtown section you'll come to the second notable shop JiCiva's Chocolates. Along the way there are plenty of other bakeries if chocolates are not of interest. Take a left onto SE 53rd Avenue and ride toward the Alberta Arts District in the northeast quadrant.

Along NE Alberta Street is Tonalli's Doughnuts and Cream where the glass case is filled with puffy sweetness. The atmosphere is vintage and the donuts melt in

your mouth. Alberta Street has many choices for other baked goods including pies at Random Order and the croissants at Petite Provence. Leave Alberta Street behind, ride along NE Vancouver Avenue and cross the Broadway Bridge into the northwest quadrant.

While there are terrific shops along NW 23rd Avenue, such as Moonstruck Chocolate, our destination is on NW Thurman Street where you'll find St. Honore Bakery. This very popular spot (there will be a line) is full of mouth-watering French pastries and the smell of brewing coffee. The 17 mile route is hardly sufficient to sample all the goodies and not compromise your figure, so plan on a return trip to sample those confections you missed the first time around.

Ride Log

0.0 Left out of Union Station and on to NW Fifth Ave towrd dowtown Portland.

0.4 Cross Burnside St and NW Fifth Ave becomes SW Fifth Ave.

0.6 Left onto SW Stark St.

0.7 Left onto SW Second Ave.

0.9 Left onto SW Ankeny St, a street closed to motor vehicles, then left onto SW Third Ave.

1.4 Left onto SW Salmon St.

1.5 Left onto SW First Ave.

1.6 Left onto SW Madison St to cross the Hawthorne Bridge; keep right where Water St exits; keep left to exit onto Hawthorne Blvd. Lower traffic streets are on block on either side of Hawthorne Blvd.

4.9 Left onto SE 53rd Ave.

5.1 Jog left at SE Taylor St to remain on SE 53rd Ave.

6.6 Left onto NE Hancock St.

7.1 Right onto NE 44th Ave.

7.2 Left onto NE Tillamook St, then right onto NE 43rd Ave.

7.6 Left onto NE Stanton St.

7.8 Left onto NE 38th Ave.

8.2 Right onto U.S. Grant Pl then right onto NE 37th Ave.

8.9 Right onto NE Klickitat St then left onto NE Alameda St.

9.1 Left to remain on NE Alameda St, then immediate right onto NE 37th Ave.

9.6 Left onto NE Going St.

9.9 Left onto NE 33rd Ave, then right onto NE Going St.

10.1 Right onto NE 30th Ave.

10.3 Left onto NE Alberta St.

10.4 Left onto NE 28th Ave.

10.6 Right onto NE Going St.

12.1 Left onto N Vancouver Ave.

13.2 Right onto NE Russell St then immediate left onto NE Flint Ave.

13.6 Right onto NE Broadway and cross the Broadway Bridge.

14.2 Right onto NW Lovejoy St immediately after crossing the bridge.

14.3 Right onto NW Ninth Ave.

14.4 Left onto NW Overton St.

15.4 Right onto NW 24th Ave.

15.7 Right onto NW Thurman St and ride under the highway.

16.2 Right onto NW 19th Ave.

16.7 Left onto NW Johnson St.

17.2 Right onto NW Ninth Ave.

17.3 Left onto NW Hoyt St.

17.4 Left onto NW Sixth Ave.

17.7 Return to Union Station. End ride.

P
P1 Voodoo Doughnuts
P2 JiCiva's Chocolates
P3 Tonalli's Doughnuts
P4 Random Order and Petite Provence
P5 St. Honore Bakery
P6 NW 23rd Ave and Moonstruck Chocolates

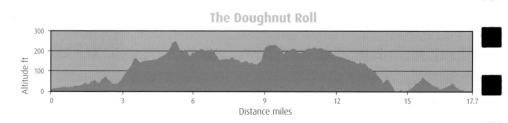

The Doughnut Roll

Altitude ft

Distance miles

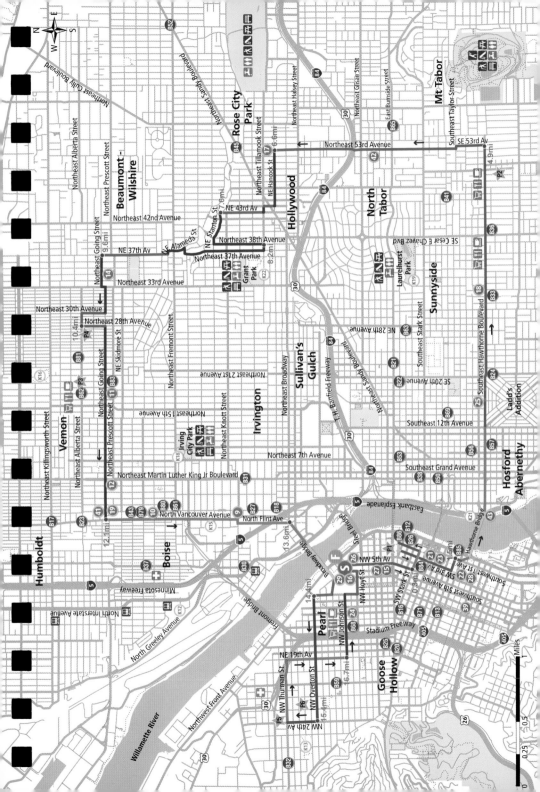

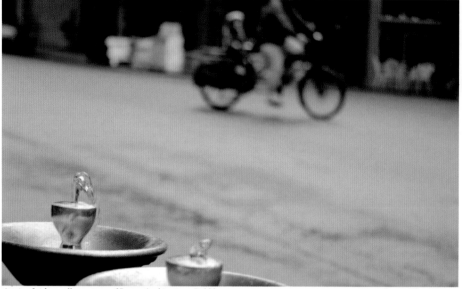

A pair of riders rolls past two of Benson's ubiquitous Bubblers.   Image Matt Wittmer

At a Glance

Distance 3.92 miles   **Elevation Gain** 320′
Distance from Downtown Portland 0.0 miles

Pioneer Courthouse Square.

Terrain
Smooth, well-maintained streets, some with train tracks.

Traffic
Moderate traffic streets through downtown Portland.

How to Get There
By car, park at any downtown garage or find on-street parking.

By public transportation, take any TriMet MAX Red or Blue line train to the corner of SW Third Avenue and SW Morrison Street. A very short walk from

Food and Drink
Lots of choices in downtown Portland for food and drinks. Restrooms are located in Pioneer Place and at Waterfront Park.

Side Trips
Mount Tabor, Rocky Butte, the East Esplanade, Laurelhurst Park, and Washington Park.

Links to 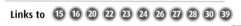 15 16 20 22 23 24 26 27 28 30 39

Where to Bike Rating

About...

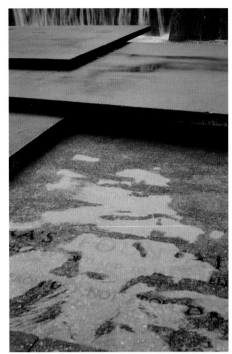

Downtown Portland is a designated Platinum City because bicycling is encouraged here. There are bike lanes, green bike boxes, and traffic signals friendly to cyclists throughout downtown. Automobile traffic is familiar with bicycles "taking the lane" to ride among the cars. This route along both city streets and bike/pedestrian paths will take you where a car cannot. Discover Portland behind the buildings and enjoy beautiful fountains along the way.

Riding up SW Third Avenue, the Ira Keller Fountain occupies an entire city block and is located across from the Keller Auditorium. On a hot summer day this fountain is the perfect place to sit on the rocks and let the spray cool you down. Continue to SW Lincoln Street to enter the Southwest Pedestrian Trail through the concrete barriers mid-way between SW First and SW Fourth avenues. On your immediate left is the Chimney Fountain, a short stack of bricks overflowing with water in the middle of the trail.

Ira's Fountain is just plain awesome. Image Matt Wittmer

Continue further down the trail through Pettigrove City Park (where you'll find The Dreamer fountain) and up to SW Fourth Avenue and SW Mill Street. This will take you to the South Park Blocks and Portland State University campus. Riding down the Park Blocks you will find several fountains including Rebecca at the Wall across from the Arlene Schnitzer Concert Hall between SW Main and SW Salmon streets. This fountain was donated by Joseph Shemanski, a Polish immigrant who became a successful businessman. The fountain includes three small, low drinking basins for dogs. Two blocks down is Director's Park where you'll find the Teachers Fountain, a recent addition to the city.

All along this ride are bowl fountains, known as Benson Bubblers. These were designed by Simon Benson, a timber baron and the owner of the Benson Hotel located on SW Broadway. The story goes that when walking the floor of one of his timber mills, he smelled beer on the breath of his workers. When asked they said there were not ready sources for fresh drinking water. To provide an alternative mid-day beverage, Benson installed 20 bowl-shaped fountains throughout the city. The consumption of beer fell by 25 percent after their installation.

The Car Wash Fountain is located at SW Fifth and Ankeny streets on your way to Waterfront Park. Here you'll find Skidmore Fountain, Portland's oldest piece of public art. One of the most interesting fountains in the city is the Bill Naito Legacy Fountain, but you won't see it if you visit during Saturday Market as it is located where the vendors set up their tents. Salmon Street Springs is the last fountain before returning to downtown.

Downtown & Theme Rides

Ride Log

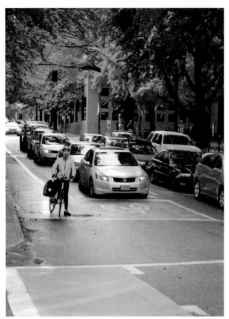

When it comes to bike boxes, color is key.
Image Matt Wittmer

P1 Ira Keller Fountain
P2 Chimney Fountain
P3 The Dreamer Fountain
P4 Arlene Schnitzer Concert Hall
P5 Rebecca at the Wall
P6 Director's Park, Teacher's Fountain
P7 Car Wash Fountain
P8 Skidmore Fountain
P9 Bill Naito Legacy Fountain
P10 Salmon Street Springs
P11 Portland Farmers Market (Saturdays)

0.0 Begin at the corner of SW Morrison St and SW Third Ave. Ride south along SW Third Ave.
0.45 Left onto SW Market St.
0.56 Right onto SW First Ave.
0.83 Right onto SW Lincoln St.
0.88 Right through the barriers mid-block onto the bike/pedestrian path.
1.12 Left around the park continuing the SW Pedestrian Trail up to SW Fourth Ave, cross via traffic light onto SW Mill St.
1.45 Right onto SW Park Ave.
2.2 Right onto SW Pine St then left onto SW Broadway, then right onto W Burnside St.
2.45 Right onto SW Third Ave.
2.5 Left onto SW Ash St.
2.66 Left onto SW Naito Parkway and ride under the Burnside Bridge.
2.8 Right onto bike/pedestrian pathway to Waterfront Bike Trail.
2.85 Right along Willamette River.
3.48 Right at Tom McCall Waterfront Park.
3.5 Right onto SW Naito Parkway then left onto SW Taylor St.
3.78 Right onto SW Fourth Ave, right through Pioneer Courthouse Square.
3.92 Return to corner of SW Morrison St and SW Third Ave. End ride.

Water Water Everywhere Fountain Ride

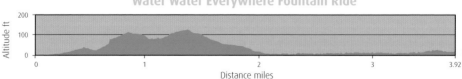

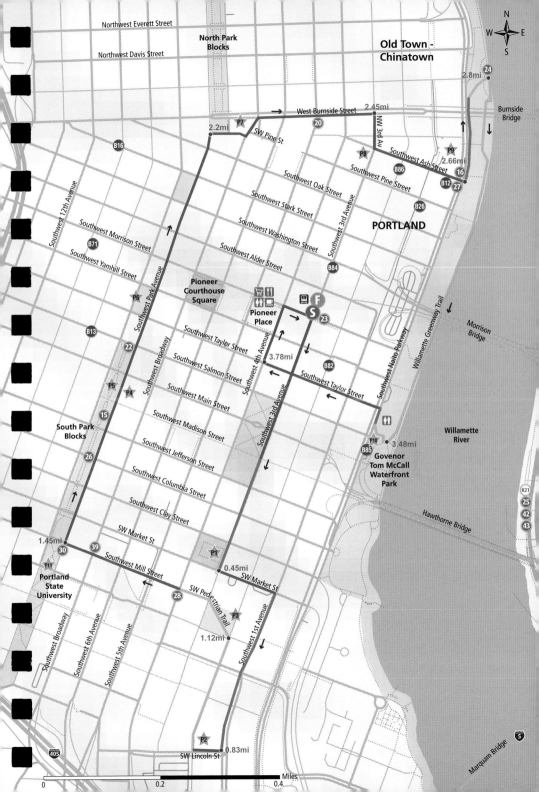

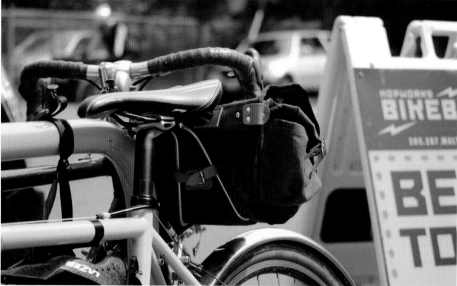

Bikes + Beers = Bikebar.

Image Matt Wittmer

At a Glance

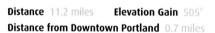

Distance 11.2 miles   **Elevation Gain** 505'

Distance from Downtown Portland 0.7 miles

Terrain

Smooth paved streets, many with bike lanes.

Traffic

Urban traffic can be heavy at commuter rush hours.

How to Get There

By car, from Pioneer Courthouse Square travel west on SW Morrison Street; left on SW 18th Avenue to the corner of SW Salmon Street. On-street parking.

By public transportation, from downtown Portland take either a Blue or Red line TriMet MAX train toward Hillsboro or Beaverton and disembark at Kings Hill/SW Salmon TriMet MAX station.

Food and Drink

Lots of opportunities for both food and drink! Public restrooms downtown Portland and at the pub of your choice.

Side Trips

Pioneer Courthouse Square, Ladd's Addition, the Laurelhurst and Irvington neighborhoods, the Alberta Arts, the Pearl, and the historic Mississippi districts are all within easy riding distance.

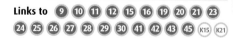

Links to 9 10 11 12 15 16 19 20 21 23 24 25 26 27 28 29 30 41 42 43 45 K15 K21

Where to Bike Rating

About...

Want to hear the heartbeat of Portland? This is the ride for you! Beer and bikes are intrinsically knit together in Portland. This relatively flat ride will let you sample both the bike and beer cultures in one spin around town. And because these locations are bike-friendly, there is always plenty of bike parking available.

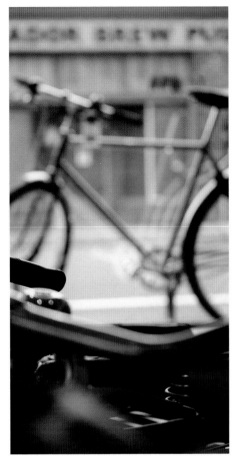

Lucky Labrador Brewpub as seen from Clever Cycles.
Image Matt Wittmer

Begin in the southwest quadrant of the city and ride through downtown Portland, over the Morrison Bridge via the cycle track. The first bike-friendly stop is Lucky Lab Brew Pub on SE Hawthorne Boulevard. There is plenty of bike parking at the rear entrance and on surrounding streets. This pub is known for its annual Tour de Lab bike race, is the launching pad for the infamous Worst Day of the Year Ride, and offers a welcoming environment for four-legged best friends. The beer is pretty good, too.

Next you will travel through the wide streets of Ladd's Addition in search of the second stop – the Apex Bar at SE 12th Avenue and SE Division Street. This is one of several pubs in the area, but is unique in having 50 beer taps and providing bike locks for cyclists with a thirst. Apex Bar offers no food, but encourages guests to bring their own. Several food establishments are located nearby.

After enjoying a beverage at Apex you'll ride along SE 12th Avenue which is somewhat narrow as you start out. Just before crossing Burnside Street a bike lane appears and provides a buffer between you and the traffic through this busy section of town. At the furthest northeast point of the ride choose one of three pubs in this bike-centric neighborhood along North Williams Avenue. Vendetta is on the corner of NE Skidmore Street and is a great choice with a backyard atmosphere. Around the corner are the Fifth Quadrant and the Hopworks Bike Bar. All three offer wonderful beer choices, ample bike parking, and outdoor seating.

Leave behind the northeast quadrant by crossing the Broadway Bridge and ride up to the Mission Theater on NW Glisan Street. This old-style theater is a terrific venue for a movie, live music, and, of course, a beer. Bike parking is a little less generous here, but there are plenty of side streets with staples to lock your bike.

These are by no means the only bike-friendly pubs in town. Use this ride to guide you and discover your favorite breweries.

Ride Log

0.0 Begin at the corner of SW Salmon St and SW 18th Ave, and ride east along SW Salmon St.

0.8 Left onto SW Second Ave.

1.0 Right onto SW Alder St and cross the Morrison Bridge.

1.5 Right onto SE Water St.

1.6 Left onto SW Salmon St.

2.1 Right onto SE Ninth Ave.

2.2 Left onto SE Hawthorne Blvd.

2.4 Right at SE 12th Ave onto SE Ladd Ave to the Ladd Circle.

2.7 Right onto SE Elliot Ave.

3.0 Right onto SE 12th Ave.

4.8 Left onto NE Lloyd Blvd, then right onto NE 11th Ave.

5.0 Left onto NE Multnomah Blvd.

5.2 Right onto NE Seventh Ave.

5.6 Left onto NE Tillamook St, jog right to cross NE Martin Luther King Blvd and remain on NE Tillamook St.

6.0 Right onto N Williams Ave.

7.1 Left onto NE Skidmore St one block, then left onto N Vancouver Ave.

8.2 Right onto N Russell St and an immediate left onto N Flint Ave.

8.7 Right onto N Broadway to cross the Broadway Bridge and continue along NW Broadway crossing Burnside St.

8.8 Right onto SW Washington St.

10.3 Right onto SW 14th Ave.

10.5 Left onto NW Glisan St.

10.8 Left onto NW 19th Ave (which becomes SW 18th Ave after crossing Burnside St) passing the Jeld-Wenn Field and returning to the corner of SW Salmon St.

11.2 End ride.

P1 Lucky Lab Brew Pub
P2 Apex Bar
P3 Vendetta
P4 The Fifth Quadrant, Hopworks Bike Bar
P5 Mission Theater
P6 Jeld-Wenn Field

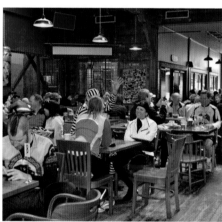

A friendly, boisterous crowd of cyclists gather in a local pub.

Bike-Friendly Brewery Tour

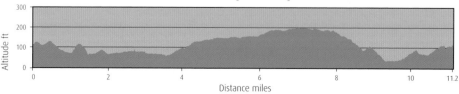

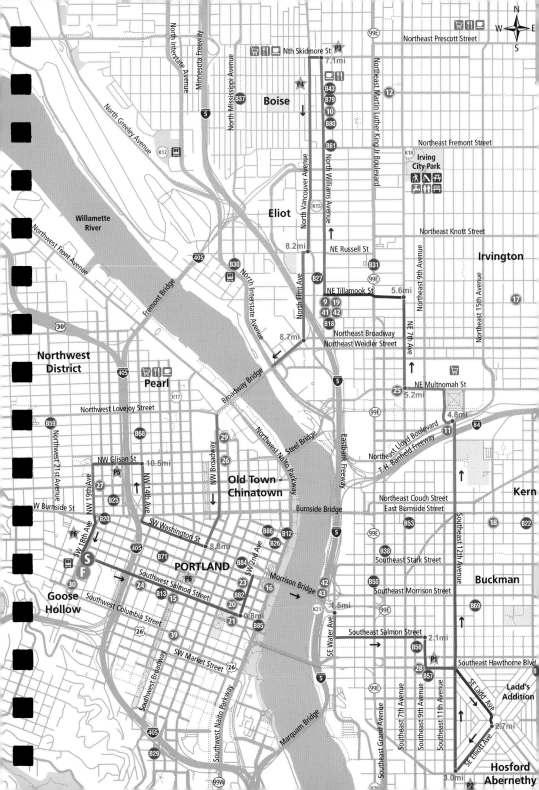

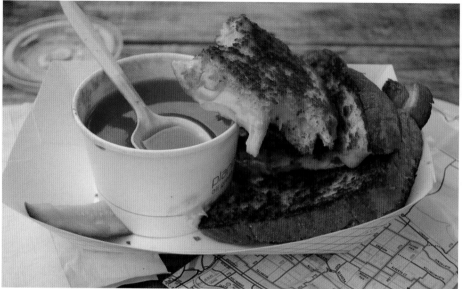

The Kindergartner, tomato soup, and pickle spear at The Grilled Cheese Grill.   Image Matt Wittmer

At a Glance

Distance 13.5 miles   **Elevation Gain** 635'
Distance from Downtown Portland 0.0 miles

Terrain

Smooth, well-maintained streets, with bike lanes and some with train tracks.

Traffic

Moderate traffic on urban streets through downtown Portland and neighborhoods.

How to Get There

By car, park at any downtown garage or find on-street parking.

By public transportation, take any red or blue line MAX train to the corner of SW Third Avenue and SW Morrison Street. A short walk from Pioneer Courthouse Square.

Food and Drink

This ride is all about finding lots of choices for food and drinks. Restrooms are located in Pioneer Place and at Waterfront Park. Some food cart pods also have facilities.

Side Trips

Downtown St. Johns, Hawthorne District, Belmont District, Historic Mississippi District, and the Alberta Arts District all have interesting food carts, restaurants, and cafés.

Links to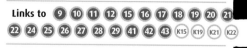

Where to Bike Rating

About...

While food cart pods abound in Portland, this ride will take you to carts voted as the very best in Portland based upon the Willamette Weekly newspaper (**www.wweek.com**) which each year features the best of Portland according to local residents. A recent count indicated that there are over 500 food carts dotted throughout the city, titled "pod profusion" by the Willamette Weekly newspaper. The variety of food available is staggering. Of course you can find the typical fried varieties, but also available are healthy choices made from fresh local ingredients.

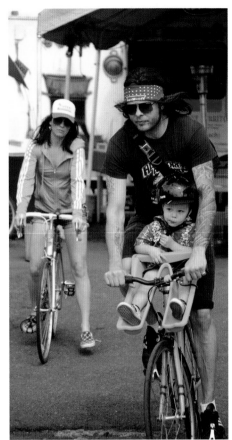

A young family exits a food pod.   Image Matt Wittmer

Begin downtown where some of the oldest food carts can be found along SW Third Avenue and SW Stark Street. Continue through Old Town and along the waterfront to cross the Steel Bridge. If you are doing this ride on the weekend you'll find a beer garden and food carts at Saturday Market. Once across the bridge you are in the northeast quadrant heading for the historic Mississippi neighborhood. On the corner of NE Skidmore Street and NE Mississippi Avenue you'll find a popular pod with plenty of bike parking on the street and an ATM in the pod. Picnic tables and tarps overhead make your visit here more comfortable.

Continue through the Mississippi District and onto NE Vancouver Avenue. There are food carts in the parking lot of a dry cleaner establishment at the corner of NE Fremont Street that you will pass on your way to NE Tillamook Street. More food carts greet you at the corner of N Williams Avenue and NE Tillamook Street. At NE 28th Avenue you'll jog left to pick up US Grant Place. This will take you to the Hollywood District where you'll cross I-84 via a bike/pedestrian bridge. The switchbacks are a bit narrow so you may

want to walk your bike. You are heading for the Belmont District where you'll find a well-established pod between NE 42nd and NE 44th avenues.

Return along bike-friendly SE Ankeny Street and cross the Hawthorne Bridge. But before you do, a visit to the small food cart on the corner of SE Seventh Avenue and SE Madison Street may be in order just to be served by one of the bikini-clad Baristas.

The Hawthorne Bridge, the oldest highway bridge in Portland, is a well-traveled bicycle route to and from downtown Portland. Bicycles travel on the outer edge of the sidewalk and pedestrians on the inside. Take this section slowly as cars, trucks and buses will be speeding past you on the steel bridge deck.

Ride Log

0.0 Begin at the corner of SW Third Ave and SW Morrison St and ride south along SW Third Ave.

0.1 Left onto SW Salmon St; left onto SW Second Ave.

0.2 Right onto SW Ankeny St, cross SW Naito Parkway, left along the Waterfront Bike Path.

0.5 Right across the Steel Bridge bike/pedestrian path, veer left up the switchbacks.

1.0 Left along NE Lloyd Blvd sidewalk to the traffic light, cross diagonally with the bike signal to take a left onto NE Lloyd Blvd. Follow the green bike lanes.

1.1 Cross NE Multnomah St onto NE Wheeler St and continue straight.

1.3 Slight right onto N Williams Ave.

2.8 Left onto N Skidmore St.

3.2 Left onto N Mississippi Ave.

3.4 Left onto N Shaver St.

3.8 Right onto N Vancouver Ave.

4.8 Left onto NE Tillamook St.

5.1 Jog right at MLK Blvd to remain on NE Tillamook St and jog right again at NE Seventh Ave to remain on NE Tillamook St.

6.3 Left onto NE 28th Ave.

6.4 Right onto NE U.S. Grant Pl.

7.2 Right onto NE 42nd Ave.

7.3 Jog right at NE Broadway to remain on NE 42nd Ave.

7.4 Cross diagonally into the bus station and cross the highway via the bike/pedestrian path.

7.6 At the end of the ramp, slight right on NE Senate St

to pick up NE 42nd Ave.

8.2 Jog slight left onto NE 41st Ave.

8.7 Cross E Burnside St and NE 41st Ave becomes SE 41st Ave.

8.9 Jog right at SE Stark St to remain on SE 41st Ave.

9.1 Jog left on SE Morrison St then right onto SE 42nd Ave.

9.2 Left onto SE Yamhill St.

9.3 Left onto SE 44th Ave.

9.4 Left onto SE Belmont St.

9.5 Right onto SE 42nd Ave, left on SE Morrison St, and right onto SE 41st Ave.

9.7 Jog right at SE Stark St to remain on SE 41st Ave.

10.0 Left onto SE Ankeny St.

11.4 Left onto SE 16th Ave.

12.0 Right onto SE Salmon St.

12.4 Left onto SE Eighth Ave.

12.5 Right onto SE Madison St and cross the Hawthorne Bridge.

13.4 Right onto SE Second Ave.

13.5 Left onto SW Morrison St to SW Third Ave. End ride.

P P1 Pod: SW Third and Stark
P2 Pod: Saturday Market, Waterfront Park
P3 Pod: Mississippi and Skidmore
P4 Pod: Vancouver and Fremont
P5 Pod: Tillamook and Williams
P6 Pod: Belmont and 42nd
P7 Pod: Seventh and Madison

Tour of the Food Carts

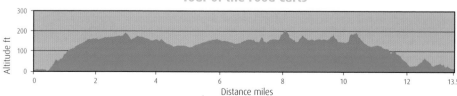

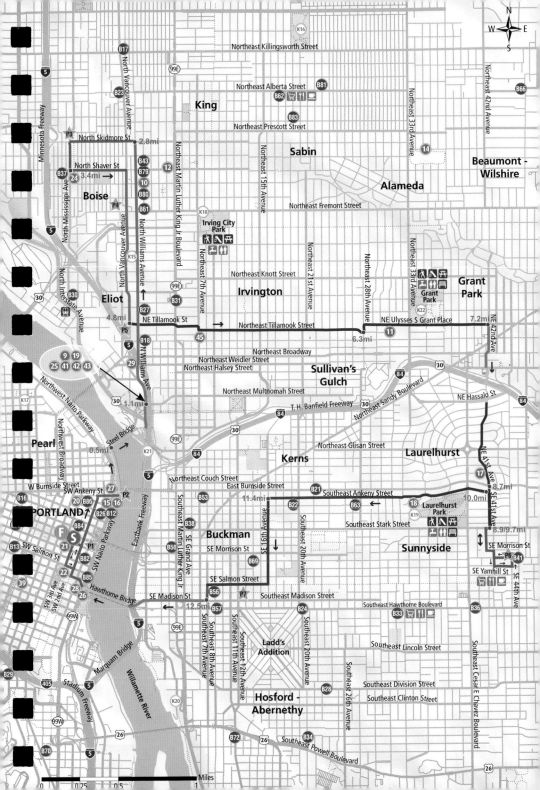

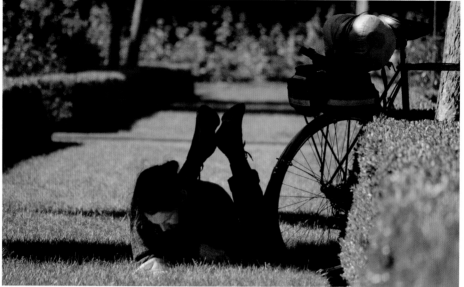

Immaculate Peninsula Park is well worth the break.

Image Matt Wittmer

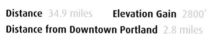
At a Glance

Distance 34.9 miles   **Elevation Gain** 2800′
Distance from Downtown Portland 2.8 miles

Terrain

Smooth, paved streets, many with bike lanes, in downtown and North Portland. Steep hills and narrow roads in the West Hills.

Traffic

Urban traffic can be heavy at commuter rush hours. Low traffic throughout the West Hills neighborhoods and up to Council Crest Park.

How to Get There

By car, take U.S. Route 26 to exit 72 toward Zoo/Forestry Center. On-street parking.

By public transportation, from downtown Portland take TriMet MAX Blue or Red line trains toward Hillsboro or Beaverton and disembark at Washington Park.

Food and Drink

There are many convenience stores, cafés and pubs located in downtown Portland. Restrooms are available between the TriMet MAX stations in Washington Park.

Side Trips

Duniway Lilac Park, George Himes Park, Council Crest, PSU campus, the Pearl District, and downtown Portland are all readily accessible.

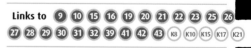
Links to 9 10 15 16 19 20 21 22 23 25 26 27 28 29 30 31 32 39 41 42 43 K8 K10 K15 K17 K21

Where to Bike Rating

About...

Matt Groening, creator of the popular television series, The Simpsons, grew up in the West Hills of Portland and named many of his characters after local streets. Take this ride to explore his childhood neighborhood and get to know both the Simpsons characters and the city in a whole new way. Challenging hills and breathtaking scenery lie ahead as you ride through urban forests, to the working waterfront, and through quaint residential neighborhoods. Character references are provided in parentheses.

The Oregon Zoo is located very near Matt Groening's childhood home and this is the starting point of the ride. He attended Ainsworth Elementary School and Lincoln High School both located in the southwest quadrant of the city. Travel up through the West Hills to the summit of Council Crest before taking the steep plunge down Montgomery Drive (Montgomery Burns, evil boss) into downtown Portland. Along the way take time to stop and look out over the five mountain peaks at Council Crest Park and marvel at the thick moss clinging to the trees along Fairmount Boulevard.

You will quickly move from urban forest to downtown commercial district and cross both NW Kearney (Kearney Zzywicz, bully) and NW Flanders (Ned Flanders, next door neighbor) streets before turning onto Lovejoy (Reverend Timothy Lovejoy). Cross the Broadway Bridge and head toward north Portland to cross N Van Houten Street (Milhouse Van Houten, Bart's best friend) before you pick up the Peninsula Crossing Trail. A short ride through the New Columbia neighborhood will bring you to N Woolsey Street.

Come back through downtown via Broadway and begin the second set of challenging hill climbs when you take a left onto Terwilliger Boulevard (Sideshow

Bob Terwilliger, evil sidekick of Krusty the Klown). More hills are ahead as you ride through the Oregon Health and Science University campus and up Marquam Hill. The lush green forest will once again surround you along Fairmount and Humphreys boulevards on your way back to Washington Park.

Under-achieving cyclists will find themselves huffing and puffing up the steeper hills at the end of this ride, but both Bart Simpson and Matt Groening would cheer on those who accept the difficult challenge of the West Hills.

Ride Log

0.0 Begin at the TriMet MAX station at Washington Park and ride down SW Knights Blvd past the World Forestry Center and the Children's Museum and continue along SW Zoo Rd.
0.4 Right onto SW Canyon Court.
1.0 Left onto the bike path at the stop sign on the corner of SW Westgate Dr and ride up to Sylvan.
1.2 Left at SW Skyline Blvd crossing the bridge and riding on the sidewalk on the opposite side of the traffic.
1.3 Cross the highway entrance ramp and SW Humphrey Blvd to continue onto SW Hewett Blvd.
3.0 Left onto SW Patton Rd.
3.1 Right onto SW Talbot Rd.
3.3 Left onto SW Talbot Terrace.
3.4 Right onto SW Greenway Ave.
3.7 Right onto SW Council Crest Dr to ride around the Council Crest summit; exit the park.
4.3 Right to continue on SW Council Crest Dr.
5.0 Left onto SW McDonnell Terrace then left onto SW Fairmount Blvd.
6.3 Right onto SW Talbot Rd then right onto SW Greenway Ave.
6.7 Left onto SW Patton Rd then right onto SW Montgomery Dr.
7.5 Jog left at SW Myrtle St to continue on SW Montgomery Dr, then jog left again at SW 21st Ave to continue on SW Montgomery Dr.

Ride Log continued...

8.7 Left onto SW 12th Ave.

9.9 Right onto NW Lovejoy St.

10.2 Left at the traffic light to cross the Broadway Bridge.

10.6 Left onto N Larrabee Ave which becomes N Interstate Ave.

11.3 Right onto N Mississippi Ave which becomes N Albina Ave.

13.0 Left onto N Ainsworth St.

14.2 Right onto N Willamette Blvd.

16.8 Right onto N Carey Blvd. Continue onto the Peninsula Crossing Trail at the corner of N Princeton St.

17.6 Right onto N Fessenden St leaving the Peninsula Crossing Trail.

18.3 Right onto N Woolsey Ave.

19.5 Left onto N Willamette Blvd.

21.0 Left to continue on N Willamette Blvd.

21.7 Right onto N Interstate Ave.

22.2 Left onto N Skidmore St.

22.9 Right onto N Vancouver Ave which becomes N Wheeler Ave after crossing Broadway, and cross the MAX tracks.

24.7 Left onto NE Interstate, cross NE Oregon St with the traffic light and continue onto the sidewalk.

24.8 Right onto the bike path at the green fence to cross the railroad tracks and ride down the switchbacks onto the East Esplanade, cross the Steel Bridge, and ride along the Waterfront Bike Trail.

26.0 Right onto bike path just before the Hawthorne Bridge up to the Hawthorne Bridge sidewalk; turn right at the top of the path onto SW Main St.

26.6 Left onto SW Broadway.

27.3 Slight left onto SW Sixth Ave at the traffic light, then right at the next traffic light to continue on SW Sixth Ave.

27.5 Left onto SW Terwilliger Blvd.

28.2 Right onto SW Campus Dr at the entrance to the Oregon Health and Science University campus.

29.0 Continue straight where SW Campus Dr becomes SW Gibbs Rd.

29.3 Left onto SW Marquam Hill Rd.

29.6 Left onto SW Fairmount Blvd.

32.0 Left onto SW Talbot Rd, cross SW Patton Rd onto SW Humphrey Blvd.

33.6 Right onto the sidewalk at Sylvan to cross the highway.

33.7 Right onto the SW Canyon Court bike path, slight right at the bottom of the hill to remain on SW Canyon Court.

34.5 Left onto SW Zoo Rd.

34.8 Left at SW Knights Blvd to return to the TriMet MAX Station.

34.9 End ride.

Please note: Bike shops are not shown on this map as the scale is too large for locations to be discernable. Please see other rides in this chapter for bike shop locations.

The Simpsons Ride

Please note: the profile for Ride 24 is depicted in 250ft vertical increments due to unusually high elevation.

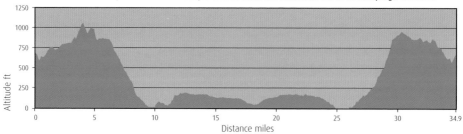

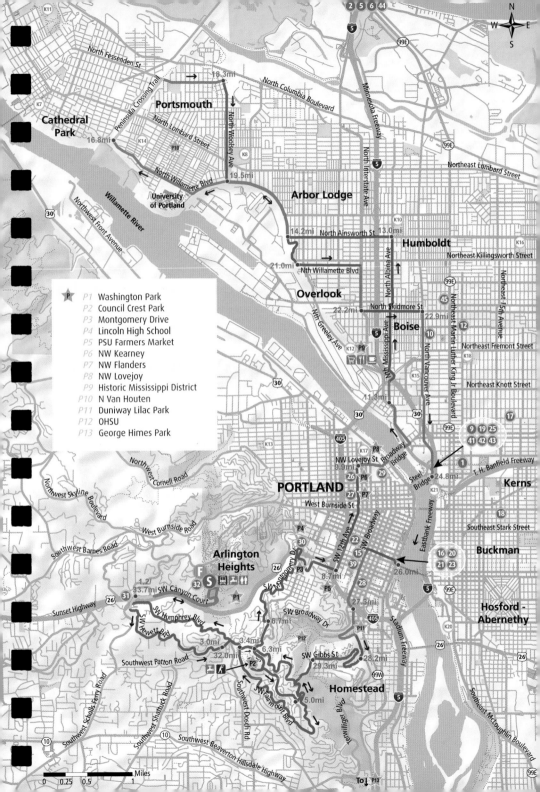

P1 Washington Park
P2 Council Crest Park
P3 Montgomery Drive
P4 Lincoln High School
P5 PSU Farmers Market
P6 NW Kearney
P7 NW Flanders
P8 NW Lovejoy
P9 Historic Mississippi District
P10 N Van Houten
P11 Duniway Lilac Park
P12 OHSU
P13 George Himes Park

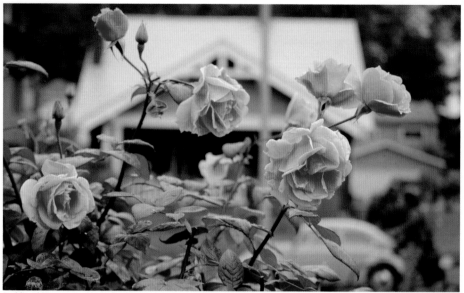

Ladd's Addition incorporates four rose test gardens and a circular central park.

Image Matt Wittmer

At a Glance

Distance 16.0 miles   **Elevation Gain** 890'
Distance from Downtown Portland 1.8 miles

Terrain

Smooth well-maintained streets and bike path.

Traffic

Urban and suburban road conditions.

How to Get There

By car, take Naito Parkway to the Steel Bridge north; left onto North Interstate Avenue. The Rose Quarter is on the left. Parking can be found either behind the Rose Quarter building on the right or on-street parking.

By public transportation, take any Red, Blue or Green TriMet MAX train to the Rose Quarter. All lines intersect at this point.

Food and Drink

There is a coffee shop at the transit center and restrooms and drinking fountains just before the Haw-
thorne Bridge on the East Esplanade and again at Crystal Springs Rhododendron Garden. Sellwood Center has numerous retail establishments.

Side Trips

Eastmoreland Golf Course, Crystal Springs Rhododendron Garden, Oak Bottom Refuge, Oaks Amusement Park and Roller Rink. Also worth a visit is Washington Park where the Japanese Garden, Hoyt Arboretum and the Oregon Zoo can be found.

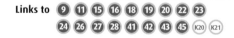

Links to 9 11 15 16 18 19 20 22 23
24 26 27 28 41 42 43 45 K20 K21

Where to Bike Rating

About...

A different view of gardens around the east side of Portland, this ride takes you through the manicured neighborhoods of Eastmoreland and the landscaped mini-gardens of Ladd's Addition. The Crystal Springs Rhododendron Garden and the Reed College campus are across from each other. Downtown Sellwood has beautiful hanging flowers and sidewalk gardens, while along the Springwater Corridor wetlands and wildflowers abound.

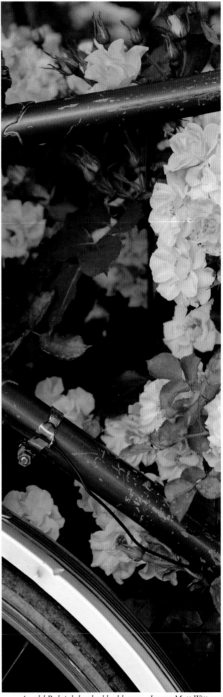

Begin at the TriMet Rose Quarter MAX Station and ride through the urban area of the Lloyd District, over I-84 and into bike-friendly neighborhoods. The streets are wide and the only real traffic you'll encounter is at busy intersections.

The Clinton Street Theater will be on your right after you turn onto SE Clinton Street. This is the location of the annual film festival, Filmed by Bike, when the cycling community comes together to celebrate bicycling, and amateur film-makers flex their creative muscle.

A bit down the road is the Crystal Springs Rhododendron Garden on the right and Reed College on the left. Both are worth a little time to explore the season's abundance of flowers. Reed College is located on a campus reminiscent of small town New England Colleges with its brick buildings and grass courtyards.

After turning at Eastmoreland Gardens onto SE 27th Avenue, your ride will take you along residential streets with beautifully landscaped homes and colorful play structures tucked between the road and the golf course. Your return trip through quaint Sellwood will bring you back to the East Esplanade via the multi-use pathway of the Springwater Corridor.

An old Raleigh backed by blooms. Image Matt Wittmer

Downtown
& Theme Rides

Ride Log

P1 Ladd's Addition
P2 Clinton Street Theater
P3 Crystal Springs Rhododendron Garden
P4 Reed College
P5 Eastmoreland Golf Course
P6 Oaks Amusement Park
P7 OMSI

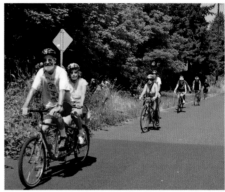

Sprinwater Corridor is a popular trail.

0.0 Starting at the Rose Quarter TriMet MAX station; right onto NE Multnomah St.

0.3 Right onto NE Seventh Ave.

0.6 Left onto Lloyd Blvd.

0.9 Right onto NE 12th Ave.

1.0 Left onto NE Irving St.

1.2 Right onto NE 16th Ave; jog left at Hawthorne St to remain on NE 16th Ave.

2.4 Ride half way around rose garden island to remain on NE 16th Ave.

2.6 Enter Ladd's Circle.

2.7 Right onto SE Ladd Ave toward Woodstock.

3.0 Left onto SE Division; immediate right onto SE 21st Ave.

3.1 Left onto SE Clinton St.

3.3 Right onto SE 26th Ave and cross SE Powell Blvd.

4.0 Left onto SE Gladstone St.

4.1 Right onto SE 28th ; cross SE Holgate Blvd.

5.1 Left into Reed College campus; ride through campus.

6.8 Left out of the campus back onto SE 28th Ave which becomes SE Tolman St and then SE Bybee Blvd.

7.3 Left at Eastmoreland Gardens onto SE 27th Ave which becomes SE Crystal Springs Blvd.

8.3 Right onto SE 37th Ave.

8.5 Right onto the Springwater Corridor Trail toward Portland.

9.5 Take a sharp right into SE 19th Ave at concrete barriers.

9.8 Left onto SE Umatilla St; cross the railroad tracks.

10.6 Right onto Springwater Corridor Trail which ends at SE Fourth Ave in an industrial area.

13.8 Left onto SE Caruthers St.

14.0 Access the East Esplanade at the end of the cul-de-sac.

15.1 Left onto the floating section of the East Esplanade.

15.6 Right onto switchbacks at Steel Bridge.

15.8 Left on sidewalk up to traffic light; cross diagonally with bike signal onto NE Lloyd Blvd.

15.9 Right onto NE Wheeler St. Follow green bike lanes.

16.0 Return to Rose Quarter TriMet MAX station. End ride.

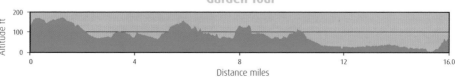

Garden Tour

Altitude ft

Distance miles

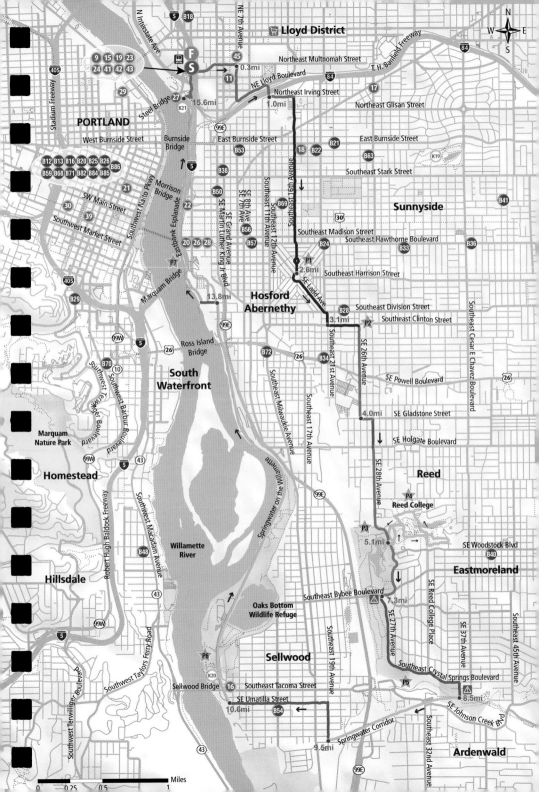

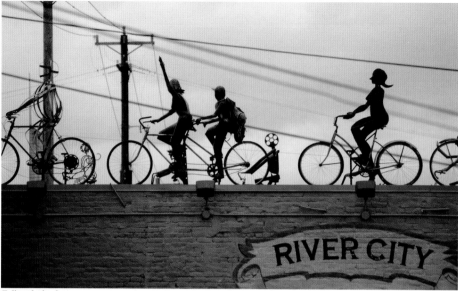

Follow the leader.

Image Matt Wittmer

At a Glance

Distance 7.1 miles **Elevation Gain** 420′
Distance from Downtown Portland 0.7 miles

Terrain

Smooth, paved, urban streets with bike lanes and bike/pedestrian paths. One short section of on-street train tracks.

Traffic

Urban traffic on streets. Bridge crossings made safer with bike-designated paths.

How to Get There

By car, from Pioneer Courthouse Square in downtown Portland, travel north on SW Sixth Avenue. This road will put you directly in front of Union Station where the ride begins. On-street parking.

By public transportation, take the TriMet MAX Green line toward Clackamas Town Center to the corner of NW Sixth Avenue and NW Hoyt Street.

Easily accessible by foot from Pioneer Courthouse

Square by walking down SW Sixth Avenue (becomes NW Sixth Avenue after crossing Burnside Street).

Food and Drink

Readily available at copious places along the ride.

Side Trip

Do the Public Art Walking Tour in downtown Portland, visit the Portland Art Museum, the Museum of Art and Craft. Monthly art-centered events include First Thursday in the Pearl District and Last Thursday in the Alberta Arts District.

Links to 9 11 15 16 19 20 21 22 23 24 25 27 28 29 30 41 42 43 45 K21

Where to Bike Rating

About...

Loop around the city to experience the beauty and culture of Portland through the lens of public art installations. Do not judge this route strictly on distance or elevation. The challenge of this ride is in seeking out art in our midst. There are many, many examples of public outdoor art in Portland and this short ride is a quick introduction to just a few.

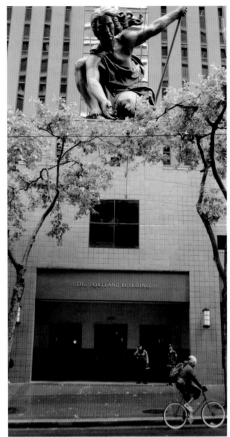

Portlandia appears to greet this passing cyclist.
Image Matt Wittmer

Begin at Union Station and ride the short distance to Jamison Square. Here you'll find "Tikitotemoniki Totems" along NW 11th Avenue. Artist Kenny Scharf built these 30-foot totems to show that art should be fun – and these four totems certainly are!

The next stop is SW 13th Avenue just after crossing Burnside Street. The "People's Bike Library of Portland," a wonderful collection of bicycles locked around a pole and topped with a small golden bicycle. This sculpture was erected by artists Brian Borrello and Vanessa Renwick in collaboration with Zoobomb (www.zoobomb.net), and is a celebration of Portland's bike culture. Travel up the SW 13th Avenue hill and find the Outside In building mural that was created by Debra Beers in collaboration with homeless youth.

Continue through downtown Portland along SW Madison Street and stop for a peek at "Portlandia" perched above the entrance of the Portland Building on SW Fifth Avenue. This, the second largest copper statue in the United States (after the Statue of Liberty), was created by Raymond Kaskey in 1985.

After crossing the Hawthorne Bridge, where you'll ride on the sidewalk, stop at the Multnomah County Building to appreciate the bronze sculpture by Wayne Chabre titled "Connections." Being located in a heavily travelled area of town, this art installation is often overlooked and deserves a closer view.

The Franz Bakery spinning loaf of bread is an example of commercial kitsch on NW 12th Avenue, which you will pass on your way to the Rose Quarter. Here you'll find "The Little Prince," an enormous crown in front of the Rose Garden Arena by Ilan Averbuch. After returning to the west side via the Steel Bridge you'll encounter "Friendship Circle" by Lee Kelly and Michael Stirling which commemorates the friendship between Portland and our sister city, Sapporo, Japan. Continue along the Waterfront Bike Trail and ride through the Old Town section past Chinatown streets on your way back to Union Station.

Ride Log

0.0 Begin at Union Station and turn left on NW Irving St.

0.1 Right on NW Fifth Ave.

0.2 Right on NW Glison St.

0.38 Right on NW Park St.

0.4 Left on NW Hoyt St then right on NW Ninth Ave.

0.57 Left on NW Johnson St past Jamison Square.

0.76 Left on NW 13th Ave, cross Burnside St and continue up SW 13th Ave.

1.67 Left onto SW Columbia St.

1.9 Left on SW Park St, also known as the South Park Blocks.

2.0 Right on SW Madison St and cross the Hawthorne Bridge.

2.8 Continue straight on SE Hawthorne Blvd.

3.47 Left onto SE 12th Ave. Make a box turn at the traffic light to turn left.

4.66 Left at traffic light onto NE Lloyd Blvd.

4.92 Right on Seventh Ave.

5.19 Left onto NE Multnomah Blvd.

5.57 Left at traffic light onto NE Wheeler Ave, cross the MAX tracks, and take a left onto NE Lloyd Blvd.

5.73 Cross NE Oregon St with the bike signal and ride onto the sidewalk; right at the green fence onto the bike path to cross the railroad tracks.

5.84 Continue down the switchbacks onto the East Esplanade and continue straight over the Steel Bridge to cross the Willamette River and ride along the Waterfront Bike Trail.

6.38 Right through the park, cross NW Naito Parkway onto NW Couch St.

P1   Jamison Park, Totems
P2   People's Bike Library
P3   Outside In
P4   Portlandia
P5   Multnomah County Building, Connections
P6   Franz Bakery
P7   The Little Prince, Rose Quarter
P8   Waterfront Bike Trail, Friendship
P9   Chinese Garden

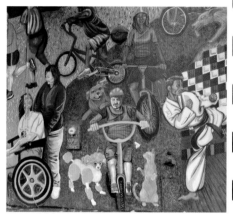

Celebrating the diversity of the Portland community, bicycles take a prominent place in this wall mural.

6.51 Right onto NW Second Ave.

6.66 Left onto NW Flanders St.

6.75 Right onto NW Fourth Ave.

6.85 Left onto NW Hoyt St, then left onto NW Fifth Ave.

6.94 Right onto NW Glisan St then right onto NW Sixth Ave to return to Union Station.

7.1 End ride.

Public Art Ride

[Altitude profile chart: Altitude ft (0–300) versus Distance miles (0–7.1)]

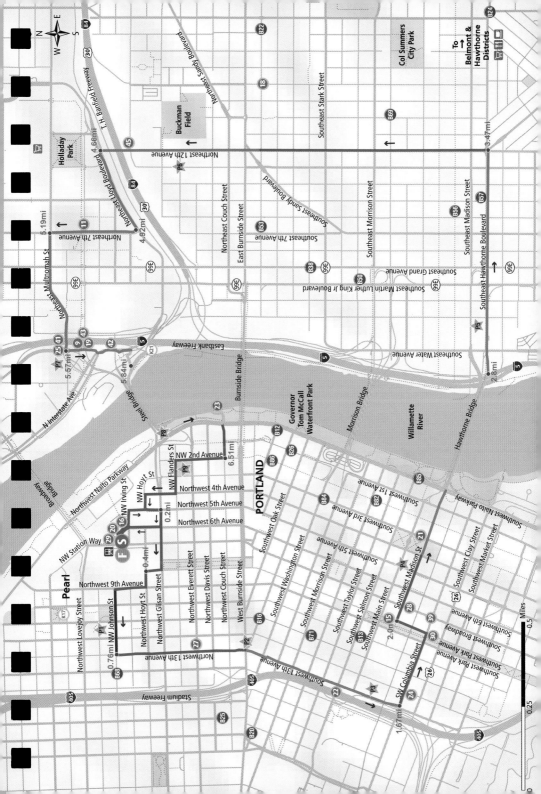

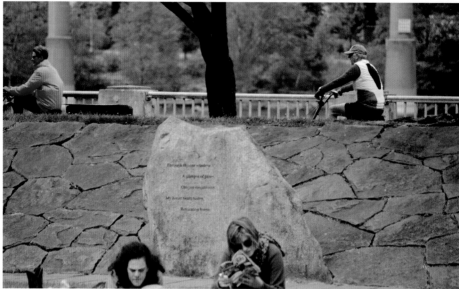

Tom McCall Waterfront Park's Japanese American Historical Plaza.

Image Matt Wittmer

At a Glance

Distance 13.0 miles   **Elevation Gain** 1614'
Distance from Downtown Portland 2.8 miles

Terrain

Smooth paved streets and bike/pedestrian trails. Switchbacks up through Washington Park are rough and have some pot holes.

Traffic

Low-traffic streets through Washington Park, bike/pedestrian trails, and urban streets with bike lanes.

How to Get There

By car, take 26 west to exit 72 toward Zoo/Forestry Center. On-street parking.

By public transportation, from downtown Portland take any Red or Blue TriMet MAX train line toward Hillsboro or Beaverton; disembark at Washington Park station.

Food and Drink

Plenty of options for food and drinks at the Rose Garden and throughout the urban parts of the ride. Restrooms available at Washington Park between the Tri-Met stations.

Side Trips

Explore NW 23rd Avenue, Oregon Zoo, World Forestry Center, the Children's Museum, the Japanese Garden, the Rose Garden, and Hoyt Arboretum.

Links to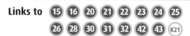

Where to Bike Rating

About...

Lots of parks, the scenic beauty being high above the city, and riding through quaint sections of town make this ride remarkable and one you will want to plan for a full-day excursion, complete with picnic lunch. This ride provides a great introduction to the city of Portland and highlights some of the most popular places to visit. Along the way you will also see some lesser known landmarks including the smallest park in the world.

Washington Park offers terrific museums and other amenities, but nothing beats riding SW Kingston Drive down through the lush, dense woods. On a summer day, listen for the whistle of the Zoo Train that may be wending its way through the forest.

Riding down this road is only half the elevation you need to descend. SW Vista Avenue is quite steep and your brakes need to be up to the task. At the bottom of the hill you're near chic NW 23rd Avenue where shopping and dining have been elevated to an art form. This area is worth a return visit.

NW Everett Street will bring you into town and along the North Park Blocks. At the corner of SW Taylor Street you'll encounter Mill Ends Park, the world's smallest park. Formerly a utility pole, this park is located in the median strip where a single evergreen tree is surrounded by a diminutive concrete wall.

Both the east and west sides of the Willamette River are parks that the public enjoys year-round. At the base of SW Ankeny Street is a wide expanse of brick and granite where fountains and parks provide terrific space for kids to play.

After crossing the Hawthorne Bridge you'll ride past Chapman Park located behind City Hall and

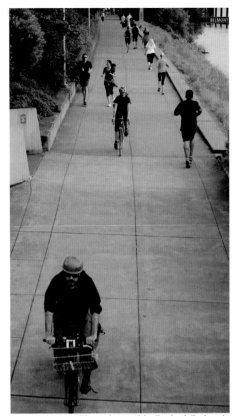

Elevated view of the Eastbank Esplanade.
Image Matt Wittmer

around the Elk Fountain in the middle of Main Street. At the top of the hill will be Shemanski Park located in the South Park Blocks across from the Portland Art Museum. Riding over SW Jefferson Street you'll come to the Jefferson Street City Park – truly more of a traffic circle than a park.

Further along at the intersection of SW 18th Avenue and Burnside Street is the Portland Firefighters Park – a park disguised as a monument. A short distance from here you will come back into the chic section of town on your way to the obscure entrance to Washington Park. You'll ride the switchbacks up to the road, through the Rose Garden access road, and ascend the remainder of the West Hills via a beautiful neighborhood along SW Fairview Boulevard before returning to the starting point.

Ride Log

P1 Rose Garden
P2 Japanese Garden
P3 NW 23rd Ave
P4 Mills End Park
P5 Chapman Park, Elk Fountain
P6 Shemanski Park
P7 Jefferson Street City Park
P8 Portland Firefighters Park

0.0 Begin at Washington Park TriMet MAX station and travel up the hill on SW Knights Blvd.

0.2 Right onto SW Kingston Dr.

1.7 Right onto SW Kingston Ave.

2.0 SW Kingston Ave becomes SW Sherwood Blvd.

2.6 SW Sherwood Blvd becomes SW Washington Way.

2.7 Right onto SW Park Place.

2.8 Left onto SW Vista Ave. Steep downhill.

3.0 Right onto NW Everett St.

4.0 Right onto NW Eighth Ave at the North Park Blocks.

4.1 Left onto NW Davis St.

4.5 Right onto NW Naito Parkway, which becomes SW Natio Parkway.

5.1 Left at SW Salmon St past the Salmon St Springs Fountain to enter the Waterfront Bike Trail.

6.0 Right to cross the N Steel Bridge via the bike/pedestrian path.

6.2 Right onto the East Esplanade.

7.3 Left up the access ramp to access the westbound side of the Hawthorne Bridge.

7.4 Right at top of ramp to cross the Hawthorne Bridge onto SW Main St.

8.2 Left at top of SW Main St onto SW Park Ave.

8.3 Right onto SW Jefferson St.

8.8 Right onto SW 18th Ave and cross Burnside St.

9.4 Left onto NW Flanders St.

9.9 Jog left then right onto NW 24th Pl.

10.0 Cross Burnside St at the traffic light to access the Washington Park entrance directly ahead. Ride up switchbacks.

10.5 Cross SW Washington Way to continue onto SW Rose Park Rd.

11.0 Right onto SW Kingston Ave.

11.2 Left onto SW Fairview Blvd.

12.6 Left onto SW Knights Blvd.

13.0 Return to Washington Park TriMet MAX station. End ride.

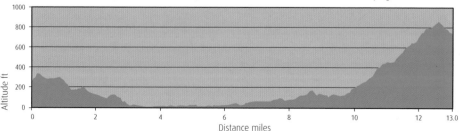

Crazy Parks Ride
Please note: the profile for Ride 27 is depicted in 200ft vertical increments due to unusually high elevation.

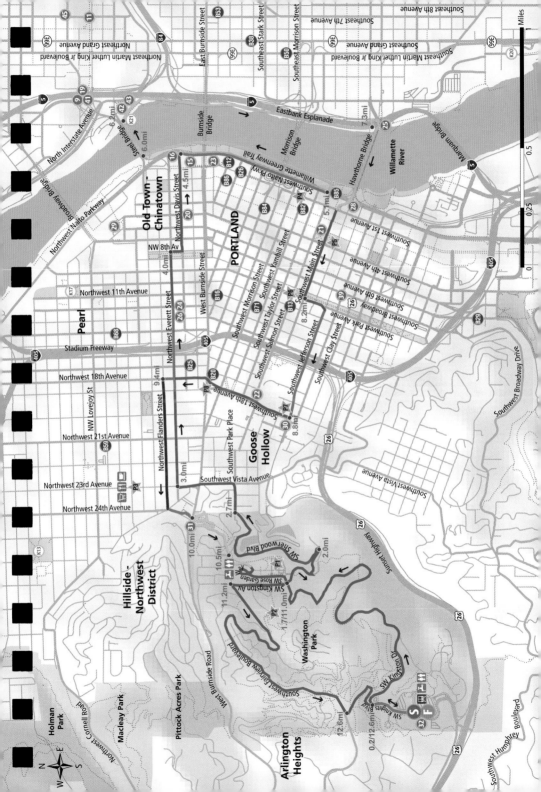

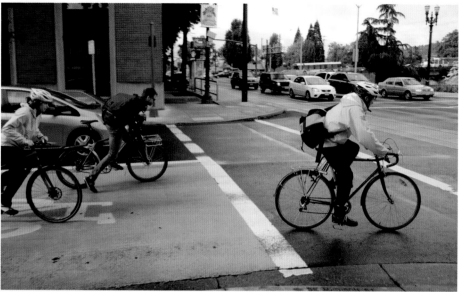

Portland consistently maintains America's highest rate of daily bicycle commuting.   *Image Matt Wittmer*

At a Glance

Distance 11.2 miles   **Elevation Gain** 665'

Distance from Downtown Portland 0.6 miles

Terrain
Smooth well-maintained streets.

Traffic
Urban, bicycle-friendly streets.

How to Get There
By car and public transportation, begin in downtown Portland on the corner of SW Harrison Street and SW Sixth Avenue, 11 short blocks southwest of Pioneer Courthouse Square. Park in one of the numerous parking stations, or on-street.

Food and Drink
There are restrooms and drinking fountains at Portland State University at the Saturday Farmers Market and numerous restaurants and cafés along the route.

Side Trip
Explore the PSU campus, the gardens in Ladd's Addition, or the Hawthorne District.

Links to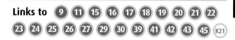

Where to Bike Rating

About...

Highlighting the bicycle infrastructure in Portland, this ride is a great introduction to the commitment the city has made to become a world-class bicycling community. Portland State University's Initiative for Bicycling and Pedestrian Innovation is a center for research focused on bicycle and pedestrian travel. By visiting **www.ibpi.usp.pdx.edu**, civic leaders — and the general public — can access studies and information about what transformed Portland into the city other communities want to emulate.

Begin this ride at the heart of Portland State University on the corner of SW Harrison Street and SW Sixth Avenue. There is ample bike parking here. I recommend doing this ride on a sunny Saturday morning so that you have an excuse to visit the farmers market at the end of your ride and enjoy the music, performances, and the abundance of fresh food and flowers available.

The route will take you down the hill to the river front and over the Hawthorne Bridge, which has over 6,000 bike commuters on a normal business day. The view of the Willamette River south shows off the marina and if you are lucky you'll see the dragon boat crews practicing on the river. To the north you'll see why Portland is known as the City of Bridges.

Down Hawthorne Boulevard are the first examples of how the city has prioritized bicycles with green bike boxes at intersections. Several of the intersections along Harrison Street have specific treatments that allow bicyclists to access roadways that prohibit motorized vehicles.

At busy intersections there are bike/pedestrian walk signals to assist in safe crossing. And one especially useful street marking is the designated left-turn lanes for bicycles only. Of course bike lanes are painted on

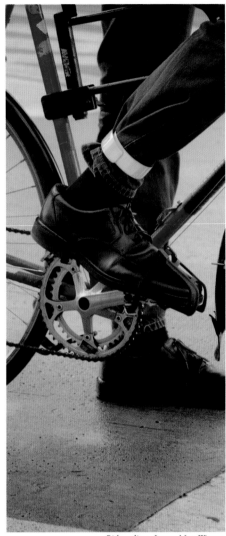

Ride to live. Image Matt Wittmer

many city streets and this ride will take you on several.

As you come to the traffic light at the intersection of NE Lombard Street and Broadway, after crossing the Broadway Bridge, notice the traffic signals. There are signals specific to cars, to bikes, and to the streetcar. This type of infrastructure allows for a variety of road use even at wide and busy intersections such as this one.

Ride Log

0.0 Begin at the corner of SW Harrison St and SW Sixth Ave and ride down the hill toward the river.

0.2 Left onto SW Fourth Ave.

0.5 Right onto SW Madison St and cross the Hawthorne Bridge ahead.

1.7 Right onto SE Ladd Ave.

2.1 Enter Ladd's Circle, ride half way around and take fifth right onto SE Harrison St.

2.2 Enter rose garden; ride half way around to continue on SE Harrison St.

2.9 Continue on SE Harrison St which becomes SE Lincoln St through the diverter.

3.1 Right onto SE 34th Ave.

3.4 Left onto SE Clinton St.

3.9 Left onto SE 41st Ave.

4.1 Left onto SE Taylor St.

5.0 Right onto SE 36th Ave.

5.1 Left onto SE Yamhill St then right onto SE 35th Ave.

5.2 Right onto SE Belmont St.

5.6 Left onto SE 42nd Ave then left onto SE Morrison St.

5.7 Right onto SE 41st Ave and dog leg right at SE Stark St to remain on SE 41st Ave.

6.2 Left onto SE Glisan St.

7.3 Right onto NE 24th Ave.

7.5 Left onto NE Oregon St.

7.6 Right onto NE 21st Ave.

8.1 Left onto NE Broadway.

11.2 Return to Portland State University. End ride.

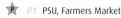
P1 PSU, Farmers Market

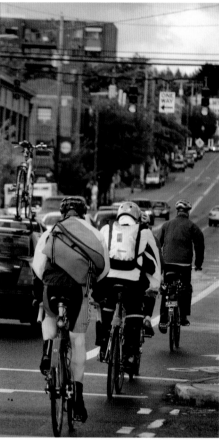
Heading home. Image Matt Wittmer

PSU to Ladd's Addition

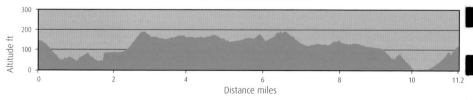

Altitude ft

Distance miles

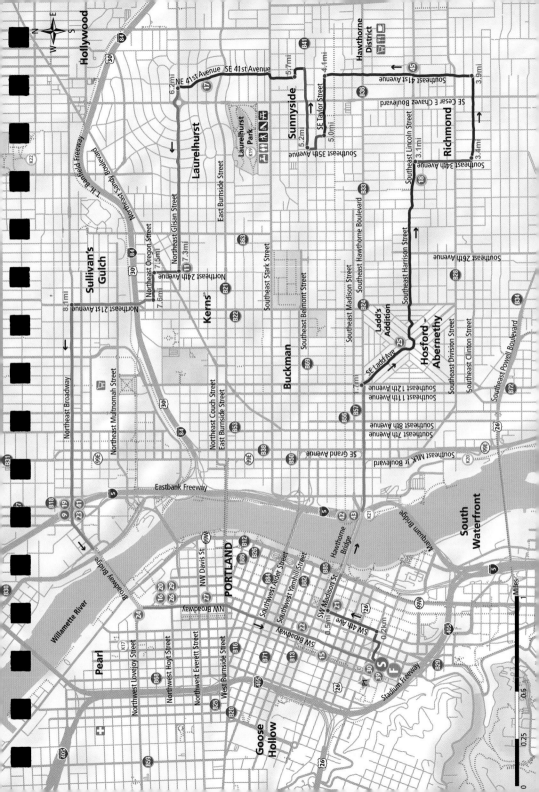

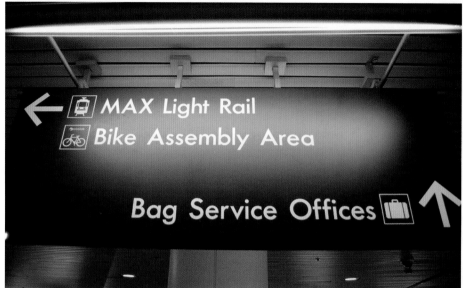

Welcome to PDX.

Image Matt Wittmer

At a Glance

Distance 10.3 miles   **Elevation Gain** 490′
Distance from Downtown Portland 0.8 miles

Terrain

Smooth, paved urban streets and neighborhood greenways with sharrows and/or bike lines on most.

Traffic

Urban streets with low to moderate traffic; bike boulevards with very low traffic, two very busy intersections.

How to Get There

By car, take SW Sixth Avenue north. The entrance to Union Station is directly ahead after crossing NW Irving Street. On-street parking.

By public transportation, take the TriMet MAX Green line toward Clackamas Town Center; disembark at NW Sixth Avenue and NW Hoyt Street.

Food and Drink

Plentiful restaurants and cafés in downtown Portland, along North Williams Avenue, and at the end of the ride at Portland airport. Restrooms and drinking fountains at Union Station and at Portland airport.

Side Trips

Whitaker Ponds Nature Park, Fernhill Park, canoe the Columbia Slough, and explore the Alberta Arts, historic Mississippi, and the Pearl districts.

Links to 5 9 10 11 12 14 16 19 20 22 23 24 26 28 41 45 K15

Where to Bike Rating

About...

One of the best ways to convince visitors that Portland welcomes bikes is to show them how to get to and from the Portland airport by bicycle. This is one of the wonderful cities where you can truly leave the automobile behind. Even with a bike fully loaded with panniers packed for faraway lands, this relatively flat ride is a great start or finish to your Portland adventure.

From Union Station ride up the hill and cross the Broadway Bridge via the sidewalk. Look to the right beyond the railroad tracks and you may see a cargo ship so large that it dwarfs the Steel Bridge.

When you take a left onto North Williams Avenue you'll be riding on a very well-travelled bike commuter route. You are in the northeast quadrant of Portland where the city boasts 25 percent ridership. Don't be surprised when you take a right onto North Going Street and find even more bicyclists on this neighborhood greenway. The recently constructed cycle track at the crossing of NE 33rd Avenue is further evidence that Portland encourages bicycle trips.

At North Holman Street ride around Fernhill Park on your way to North 42nd Avenue. This is a difficult crossing because of the fork in the road to the left which creates two converging roads of vehicles coming toward you. Thankfully there is relatively light traffic most of the time. The road is rough along this section. With the Columbia Slough (pronounced "slew") on your right you'll ride past an industrial park with wide roads and little weekend traffic. Off to the left you will see the airport control tower and you'll know you are getting close. Be sure to take a moment and look at the cannons and vehicles as you pass the Oregon National Guard. Lots of blackberry bushes grow around the slough and

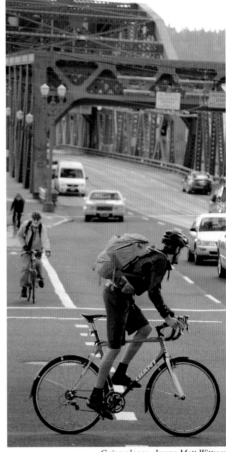

Going places. Image Matt Wittmer

provide a tasty snack in late summer.

Turning left onto NE 82nd Avenue may require a box turn to cross safely. A short distance ahead is NE Airport Way/Frontage Road. Cross all the lanes to turn left toward the airport which is straight ahead. You will see the bike path travels into the lower level of the terminal. Do not go up the access ramp. As you enter the terminal area, bike parking is on your left. There is more bike parking at the other end of the terminal and around the corner from the bike staples, there is a bike stand. The airport has tools if you need to assemble or disassemble your bike. Instructions for borrowing tools are posted on the wall. Welcome to Portland!

Downtown & Theme Rides

Ride Log

0.0 Begin at the Union Station.

0.1 Exit the station; right on NW Irving St, uphill and cross the Broadway Bridge.

0.9 Left onto N Williams Ave.

2.5 Right onto NE Going St.

4.2 Dog leg left onto the cycle track to cross NE 33rd Ave, then right to remain on NE Going St.

4.7 Left onto NE 37th Ave and cross N Killingsworth St.

5.3 Right onto N Holman St and circle around Fernhill Park.

5.5 Left onto N 42nd Ave to cross the narrow bridge; cross over NE Columbia Blvd at the traffic light. Once across NE Columbia Blvd, the road becomes NE 47th Ave.

6.4 Right onto NE Cornfoot Rd at the stop sign at the end of NE 47th Ave.

7.9 Left onto NE Alderwood Rd.

8.4 Left at NE 82nd Ave by making a box turn.

8.9 Left across the tracks and access NE Airport Way/ Frontage Rd.

9.3 Jog left at stop sign and access the bike lane/path along NE Airport Way.

10.0 Enter the terminal area.

10.3 End ride.

Please note: Bike shops are not shown on this map as the scale is too large for locations to be discernable. Please see other rides in this chapter for bike shop locations.

 P1 Mississippi District
P2 Alberta Arts District
P3 Whitaker Ponds Nature Park
P4 Oregon National Guard

Bike lane on Cornfoot Road. Image Matt Wittmer

Downtown Portland to the Airport

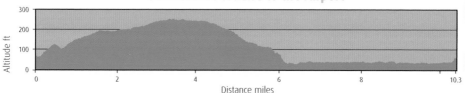

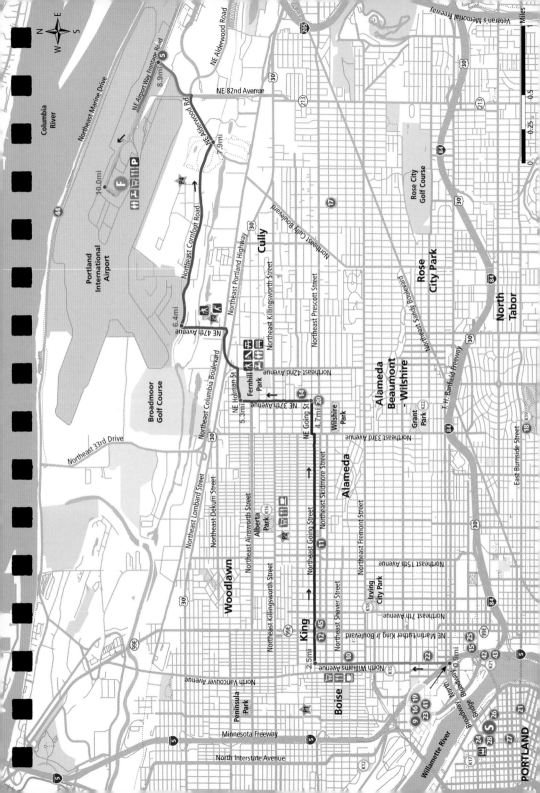

West

West of the city offers the opportunity for cyclists to challenge themselves with both distance and hills. These rides are worth the challenge, however, when you are rewarded with stunning views of the city, mountains, farmland, and vineyards. Western Oregon has climate conditions that are perfectly suited to the production of world-class wines of the Pinot Noir variety. Visitors to the region will find it fun to head southwest in search of these vineyards. Closer to downtown the hills on the west side of Portland provide access to amazing views.

The West Hills of Portland are both beautiful and challenging. Situated in the southwestern portion of the city, the summits provide magnificent vistas of distant snow-capped mountains. Some of the incline angles exceed 10 per cent, which is challenging even for the fittest cyclist, and it is recommended that you adopt a slow and steady pace if you want to reach the peak without having to dismount. Accepting the fact that some hills are just too steep is no embarrassment, and many a cyclist has been known to walk up sections of the West Hills in order to enjoy the view from the top.

Though these rides furthest west are at a distance from downtown Portland, public transportation provides easy access to the starting points. More ambitious cyclists will also find bicycling routes from downtown Portland through one of the many bicycling maps available online and in stores. In less time than you would imagine you can go from urban center to rural farmland by choosing one of the Hillsboro rides where many cyclists head on summer weekends. Even with the popularity of this area you will often find yourself alone on rural roads.

The distance and hills should not be deterrents for cyclists of less than expert skill. A sense of adventure and a curious nature are all that is required to enjoy these rides.

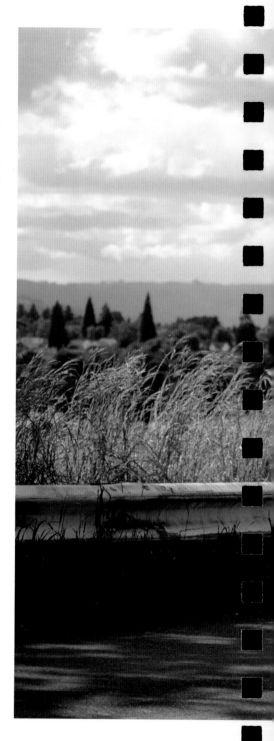

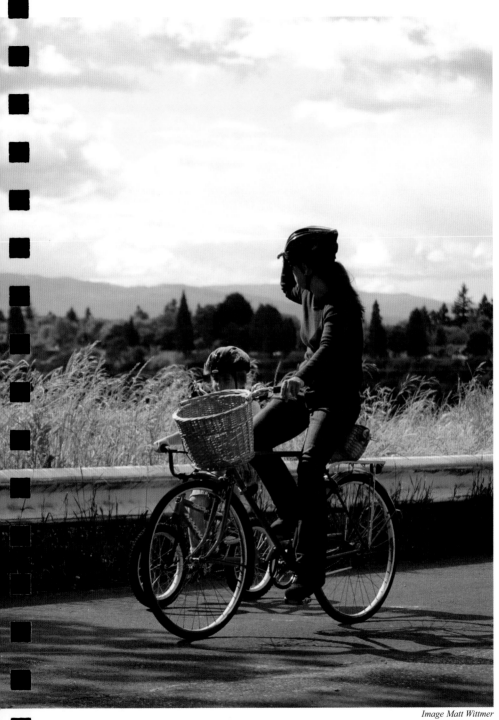

Image Matt Wittmer

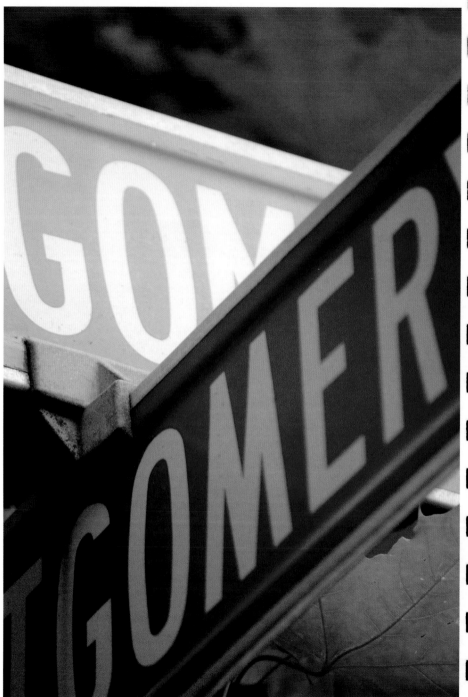

Image Matt Wittmer

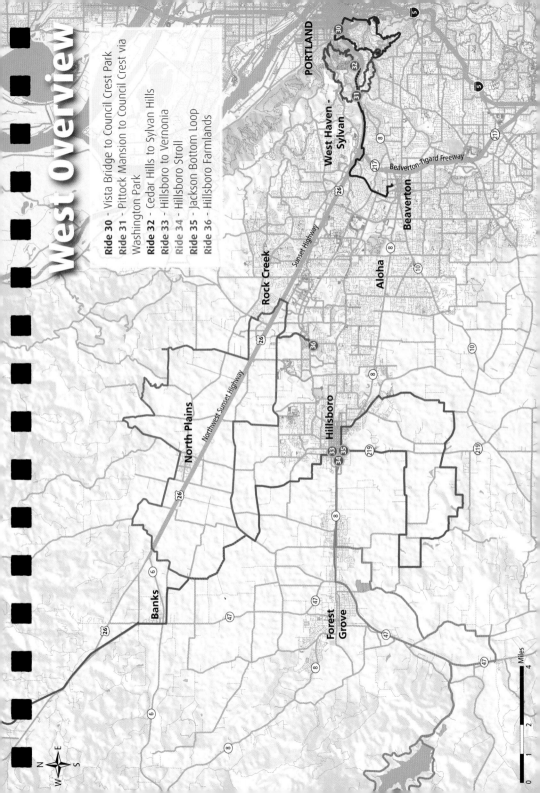

West Overview

Ride 30 - Vista Bridge to Council Crest Park
Ride 31 - Pittock Mansion to Council Crest via Washington Park
Ride 32 - Cedar Hills to Sylvan Hills
Ride 33 - Hillsboro to Vernonia
Ride 34 - Hillsboro Stroll
Ride 35 - Jackson Bottom Loop
Ride 36 - Hillsboro Farmlands

PORTLAND

West Haven - Sylvan

Beaverton

Beaverton-Tigard Freeway

Aloha

Sunset Highway

Rock Creek

North Plains

Northwest Sunset Highway

Hillsboro

Banks

Forest Grove

N
W   E
S

Miles
0   1   2   4

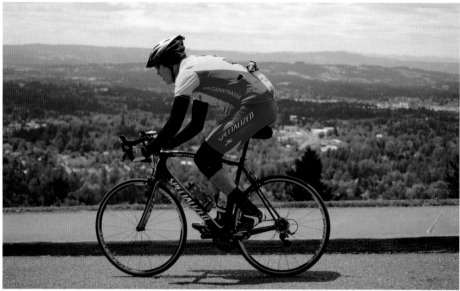

You haven't truly seen Portland until you've climbed Council Crest.

Image Matt Wittmer

At a Glance

Distance 9.7 miles   **Elevation Gain** 1538'
Distance from Downtown Portland 1.3 miles

Terrain

Paved streets, some bike lanes.

Traffic

Quiet residential neighborhoods, narrow streets. Traffic becomes heavier in downtown Portland.

How to Get There

By car, take SW Broadway, right onto SW Taylor Street, left onto SW Ninth Avenue. Continue onto SW Park Avenue and right onto SW Jefferson Street. Goose Hollow MAX station is at the bottom of the hill. On-street parking.

By public transportation, from downtown Portland take any TriMet MAX Red or Blue line train toward Hillsboro or Beaverton or any bus traveling along Jefferson Street.

Food and Drink

The popular Goose Hollow Inn is located at the start and end of your ride. There are drinking fountains at the summit of Council Crest, but no restrooms. A plethora of food and drink are available at Saturday Farmers Market.

Side Trip

Duniway Lilac Park is a great location for a picnic on your return to downtown Portland. On SW Jefferson Street is the Portland Art Museum and the Oregon Historical Society, both of which are well worth a visit.

Links to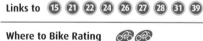

Where to Bike Rating

About...

This ride will take you through some terrific residential neighborhoods to the highest point in Portland and through two campuses before bringing you back to the Goose Hollow MAX station. You'll travel through the campus of the Oregon Health and Science University built on the hillside, and then through Portland State University campus.

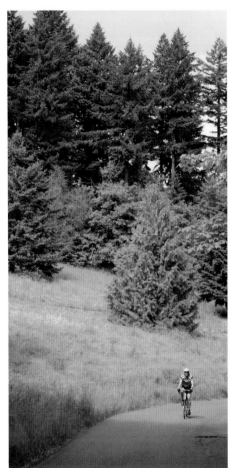

Dwarfed in a sea of green.   Image Matt Wittmer

West

The summit of Council Crest is well worth the hill climb where you get a breath-taking view of Portland and surrounding areas on a clear day. Council Crest is thought to be the highest point in Portland and boasts a fabulous view of the city and of five mountain peaks in the Cascade Range — Mounts Hood, St. Helens, Adams, Jefferson, and Rainier. Be sure to read the inscription that circles the summit to learn about the history of this location.

The ride both up to and down from the park has some interesting sights. Many of the homes in this neighborhood are built on stilts and sit precariously on the hillside. Some require stairs or bridges for street access but are valuable for their unique architecture and view of the city.

On the day of our ride the weather was foggy and damp which made the hill climb easier but robbed us of the view of the Cascade Mountain Range at the top. I especially enjoy the view from the height of the Vista Bridge because the buildings downtown seem so close from this vantage point.

On a spring day, the fragrance from the lilac bushes at the Duniway Lilac Park on SW Terwilliger Boulevard is almost intoxicating. This little park is a gem

in this part of the city. Riding into downtown Portland can be unnerving as you weave among the cars on SW Sixth Avenue, so a diversion through the campus of Portland State University is a great way to avoid the traffic. I highly recommend taking the time to stop and walk through Saturday Farmers Market. The variety of fruits, vegetables, honey, salmon, eggs, lambs, goats, and flowers is hard to imagine. Not only is there an abundance of high quality food available, but there are food carts and musicians who make the weekly event a must whenever I am close to the area on Saturdays.

Ride Log

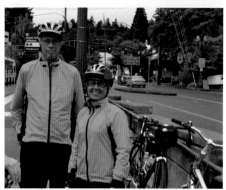

These riders are happy to be setting out on their ride even when the weather is less than ideal.

0.0 Start at the Goose Hollow MAX station and travel south on SW Jefferson St toward the Vista Bridge.

0.1 Right onto SW 20th Ave.

0.2 Left onto SW Main St.

0.3 Dog leg right at SW King Ave to remain on SW Main St.

0.4 Left onto SW Vista Ave. Cross the Vista Bridge directly ahead.

0.8 Right onto SW Montgomery Dr; this road takes a couple of turns that are easy to miss where other streets connect. Montgomery turns to the right at SW 21st Ave and turns right again at SW Myrtle St.

2.0 Left onto SW Patton Rd. Ride one block.

2.1 Right onto SW Greenway Ave. Hug the curb next to the wooden sidewalk and do not be confused when a couple of other streets join SW Greenway Ave.

2.7 Continue straight onto SW Council Crest Dr. Ride the sidewalk to enter the summit that is surrounded by a short stone wall. Leave the summit via the same sidewalk and exit the park to the right down SW Council Crest Dr to the stop sign.

3.4 Left onto SW Greenway Ave.

3.7 Left onto SW Talbot Terrace.

3.9 Sharp left onto SW Fairmount Blvd at the stop sign.

6.2 Right onto SW Marquam Hill Rd. This road turns into SW Gibbs St. Ride through the OHSU campus.

7.1 Right onto SW Campus Dr.

7.9 Left onto SW Terwilliger Blvd at the stop sign and leave the OHSU campus.

8.1 Right to continue on SW Terwilliger Blvd where SW Sam Jackson Park Rd meets Terwilliger at the traffic light and head toward downtown Portland. At SW Sheridan St, Terwilliger becomes SW Sixth Ave. Ride down the hill into downtown Portland keeping to the left lane.

8.8 Left onto SW Harrison St through Portland State University campus.

8.9 Right onto the South Park Blocks through the campus.

9.2 Left onto SW Jefferson St.

9.7 At the bottom of the hill, return to the Goose Hollow MAX station. End ride.

 P1 Portland State University

Vista Bridge to Council Crest Park

Please note: the profile for Ride 30 is depicted in 250ft vertical increments due to unusually high elevation.

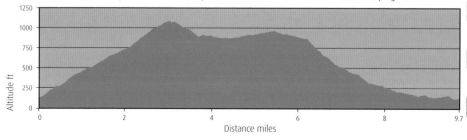

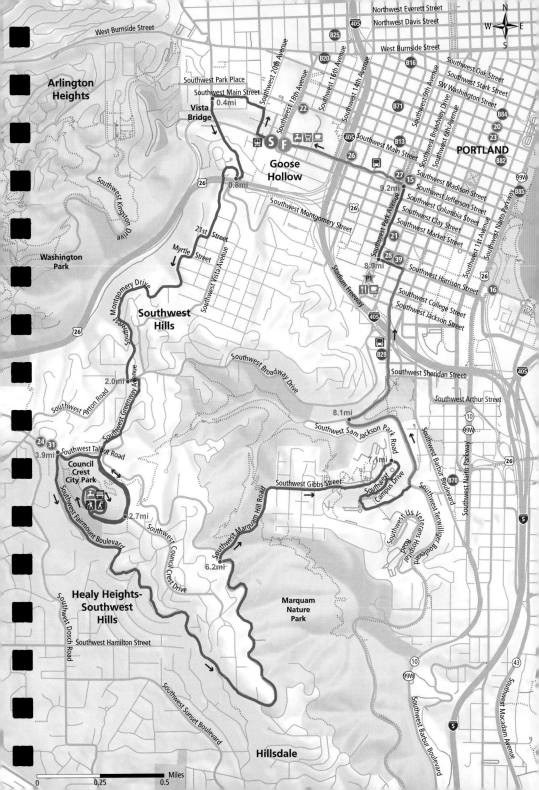

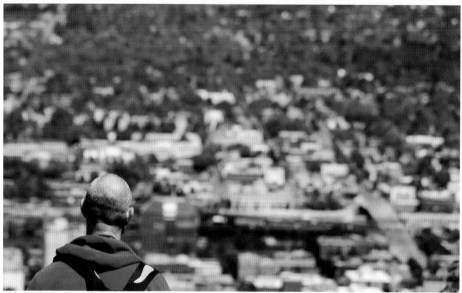

Pittock Mansion is a spot worth pondering.   Image Matt Wittmer

At a Glance

Distance 14.0 miles   **Elevation Gain** 2369′
Distance from Downtown Portland 4.5 miles

Terrain

Paved road and bike paths. Some are rough with steep descents.

Traffic

One busy crossing and low-traffic streets.

How to Get There

By car, take Exit 71B off US 26 West; right onto Skyline Boulevard, left onto SW Montgomery Street, left onto SW 58th, continue straight to SW 61st Drive. On-street parking.

   By public transportation, take Bus #58 toward Beaverton to Sylvan Hills or take the MAX train to Washington Park and ride down to Sylvan Hills. Access the SW Canyon Court from the bike/pedestrian path down the hill toward Beaverton. Take a right at the cut out in the concrete wall. Go right up the hill and find SW 61st Drive on the left.

Food and Drink

Restaurants and cafés at Sylvan Hill, and again in the NW 23rd Avenue area about a block from the entrance to Washington Park. Drinking fountains at Council Crest and restrooms at Washington Park and Pittock Mansion.

Side Trip

NW 23rd Avenue has interesting restaurants and boutiques; Pittock Mansion and the grounds; Washington Park has the Hoyt Arboretum, the Children's Museum and the Oregon Zoo. Down the hill from Washington Park are the Japanese Garden, the International Rose Garden, and monuments to the Holocaust and the Vietnam War.

Links to (24) (27) (30) (32)

Where to Bike Rating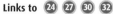

About...

This ride will take you to three of the highest points in Portland. Pittock Mansion sits about 1,000 feet above sea level and is a great place for bird watching. Washington Park is a very popular place for its museums, the Oregon Zoo, and gardens. And the highest peak in Portland is found at the summit of Council Crest Park where five mountain peaks can be viewed. Each of these locations has numerous hiking trails where you can wander through the beautiful Oregon woods.

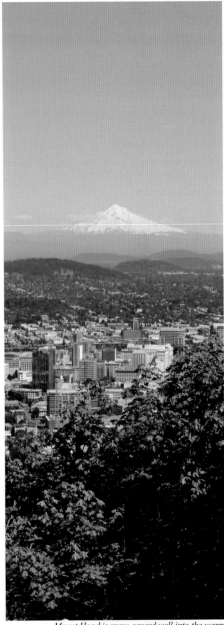

Mount Hood is snow-coverd well into the warm weather months.

The 22 room Pittock Mansion was built on 46 acres of land as the private home of the publisher of The Oregonian newspaper, Henry Pittock. His wife, Georgiana, is known as one of the founders of the Portland Rose Festival that takes place each June. The mansion and grounds receive over 80,000 visitors each year and has been featured in several movies including *Unhinged, Body of Evidence*, and *First Love*. The tree canopy provides welcome shade on a hot summer day as you slowly ascend. However, the ride downhill is terrific and provides great views of the beautiful homes, surrounding urban woods, and downtown buildings.

The second peak of the ride is at Washington Park where the extremely popular Oregon Zoo is located. The zoo is well known for its elephant husbandry program and these stately beasts have a prominent position among the other animals. The ride up to Washington Park begins with a very steep section of road and then levels off a bit.

As you descend the hill from Washington Park, you will be able to see the red and white tower that sits atop Council Crest, the next and highest peak of this ride. From the summit you can view five snow-capped mountain peaks and 3,000 miles of land. Council Crest Park is a great place for the view of the city, the mountains, and for picnicking on the grassy hillside.

West

Ride Log

0.0 Begin at SW 61st Dr.

0.7 Right onto SW Barnes Rd. At Burnside, SW Barnes becomes NW Barnes.

2.0 Left onto NW Pittock Ave and ride up the hill.

2.2 Right onto NW Pittock Dr.

2.5 Left into Pittock Mansion.

2.8 Exit the mansion grounds; left onto NW Pittock Dr which becomes NW Montevilla Ave accessible only to pedestrians and bicycles.

3.1 Left onto SW Hermosa Blvd.

3.3 Right onto NW MacLeay St.

4.0 Left onto Burnside St using the pedestrian traffic light and ride via the sidewalk down to NW 24th Ave; right into Washington Park through the gated pathway; ascend the hill via the switchbacks.

4.8 Cross at Stearns Dr and Washington Way and continue up the hill.

4.9 Cross at Wright Ave and Park Pl and follow the signs to the International Test Rose Garden.

5.3 Ascend Kingston Dr up to Washington Park.

6.8 Left onto SW Knights Rd (this becomes SW Zoo Rd).

7.4 Right onto SW Canyon Court.

8.0 Left onto the bike pathway to the Sylvan Hill traffic light.

8.2 Left over the bridge to cross SW Scholls Ferry Rd via the sidewalk.

P1 Pittock Mansion
P2 International Rose Garden
P3 Washington Park
P4 Council Crest City Park

8.4 Right onto SW Hewett Blvd.

10.1 Left onto SW Patton Rd at the stop sign; cross SW Dosch Rd.

10.2 Right onto SW Talbot Rd.

10.3 Continue straight onto SW Talbot Terrace. SW Talbot Rd veers slightly to the left but SW Talbot Terrace is straight ahead.

10.4 Right at Greenway Ave and enter Council Crest Park.

10.9 Right around the summit.

11.2 Exit the park via the road where you entered.

11.4 Left at SW Greenway Ave.

11.7 Left onto SW Talbot Terrace; this becomes SW Talbot Rd.

12.0 Continue straight across SW Patton Rd to SW Humphrey Blvd.

13.4 Right onto the sidewalk at the junction of SW Humphrey Blvd and SW Hewett Rd to the traffic light at Sylvan Hill; cross the bridge.

13.5 Left at the traffic light to the SW Canyon Court bike path.

13.9 Right onto SW Canyon Court at the cut through.

14.0 Return to SW 61st Dr. End ride.

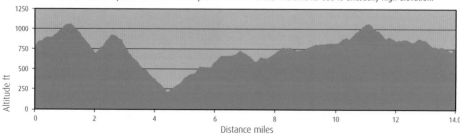

Pittock Mansion to Council Crest via Washington Park

Please note: the profile for Ride 31 is depicted in 250ft vertical increments due to unusually high elevation.

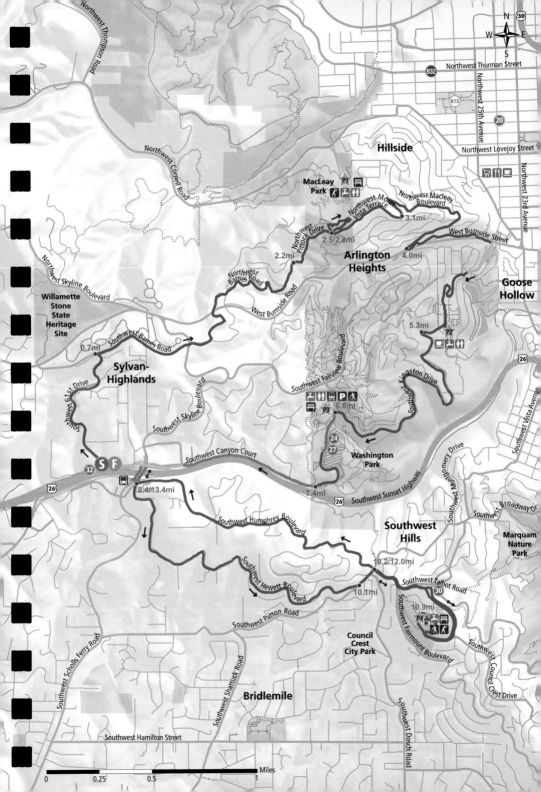

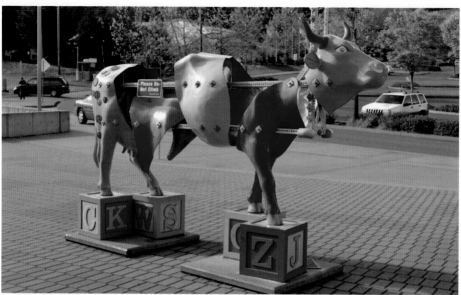

Colorful cow sculpture greets visitors at the Children's Museum.

At a Glance

Distance 6.7 miles   **Elevation Gain** 430′

Distance from Downtown Portland 6.6 miles

Terrain

Bike path, paved streets and bike lanes.

Traffic

Very limited traffic until Cedar Hills Boulevard where there are three difficult connections navigating to the Beaverton Transit Center.

How to Get There

By car, take U.S. 26 west to exit 714 to merge onto SW Canyon Road, turn right onto SW Lombard Avenue to Beaverton Transit Center MAX station. On-street parking.

    By public transportation, from downtown Portland board the TriMet MAX Red line toward the airport or the Blue line toward Gresham.

Food and Drink

There are restrooms at Washington Park, and numerous places to purchase snacks, water, and other supplies in several shopping centers along Cedar Hills Boulevard and at the Beaverton Transit Center. There are restrooms and drinking fountains along Cedar Hills Boulevard at the public parks.

Side Trip

Oregon Zoo, World Forestry Center, Children's Museum, Hoyt Arboretum, Japanese Garden, and the International Rose Garden.

Links to

Where to Bike Rating

When traveling from Washington Park to Cedar Hills Boulevard, or   in the opposite direction.

About...

In one direction this is an exhilarating downhill ride from beautiful Washington Park to the shopping centers of Cedar Hills Boulevard along a car-free bike path that parallels. Taking the route in the opposite direction provides a great hill climbing training ride up to Washington Park at the top of the West Hills where the Oregon Zoo, the World Forestry Center, Hoyt Arboretum, and the Children's Museum are located. The bike path is wide and separated from both the residential areas on one side and the highway on the other. Expect to find cyclists of all ages using this bike path as their preferred way to avoid the street traffic of alternative routes.

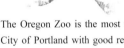

The Oregon Zoo is the most visited attraction in the City of Portland with good reason. It is home to one of the most successful elephant breeding programs in the nation. In a recent renovation, the zoo added an entire African animal exhibit. There is a train that travels around Washington Park through the woods and makes one stop down the hill at the International Rose Garden and the Japanese Garden. One train ticket pays for the two-way trip. The Zoo Lights exhibit at Christmas time is a breath-taking extravaganza of lights and music, not to be missed.

Directly across the street from the MAX station elevator is The World Forestry Center. Known for its forests, Oregon's relationship to trees and their benefits is highlighted in the exhibits at the World Forestry Center. Be sure to visit the train around the corner from the entrance to the exhibits.

The Children's Museum is just down the way from both the Zoo and the Forestry Center. Bright colors and an artistic sculpture of a cow greet young visitors at the entrance to the museum. Up the hill is the 187 acre Hoyt Arboretum with miles of hiking trails through lush forests. This park was established in 1928 to protect endangered species. The Arboretum contains more than 5,800 specimens from around the world. Hoyt Arboretum is a living laboratory where anyone can enjoy the trees and plants. Be sure to visit the information center to pick up trail maps.

This area is beloved by Portlanders and is also a favorite of the infamous Zoo Bombers. These speed-loving daredevils on bikes and long boards take the MAX train from the Goose Hollow one stop to the Washington Park station where they throw caution to the wind, defy gravity, and "bomb" down the hill.

At the other end of the ride is Cedar Hills Boulevard, which has numerous shopping centers. Several restaurants, fast food establishments, grocery stores, and other retail stores populate this area. And in between there are a cemetery and three large parks with restrooms and drinking fountains.

West

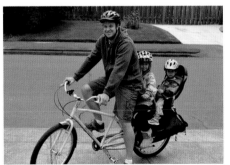

Transporting kids around the neighborhood is better by bike...

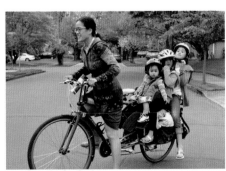

even for entire families!

Ride Log

0.0 Start at Beaverton Transit Center by taking either the Red line to the airport or Blue line to Gresham. Disembark at the Washington Park station. Take the elevator up to the park from the station.

0.4 Begin downhill on the SW Knights Blvd from MAX station which becomes SW Zoo Rd. Just before the bridge that crosses over Rte 26, also known as Sunset Hwy take a right onto SW Canyon Court.

1.0 At the top of the hill, cross over street onto bike path at SW Westgate Dr.

1.2 At the top of the hill, cross SW Skyline Blvd and access the bike path.

1.9 At SW Camelot Court take a left at the Sunset Hills Memorial Park to cross over the highway.

2.0 Take an immediate right onto SW Pointer Rd.

2.2 At SW 75th, Pointer Rd ends; access the bike path (also known as SW Park Way) to the right along the stone wall that separates the path from the Sunset Hwy.

3.2 The path ends at SW Knollcrest Rd.

3.3 Continue straight and take a left onto SW 96th Ave one block.

3.37 Right onto SW Wilshire St; cross the bridge and continue straight.

3.8 Right onto SW Marlow Ave which becomes SW Butner Rd as it curves left in front of the Sunset Transit Center.

4.5 Left onto SW Cedar Hills Blvd. An alternate starting point of this ride is at Church of Christ on the corner of SW Park Way and SW Cedar Hills Blvd where there is a TriMet Park and ride parking lot.

6.1 Left onto SW Hall Blvd.

6.3 Left onto SW Center St.

6.5 Right onto SW Lombard Ave.

6.7 Left into the Beaverton Transit Center and end of ride.

Note: This ride can be done in either direction. Going from Cedar Hills Boulevard up to Washington Park is a great training ride uphill along a wide smooth bike path. It is an exhilarating downhill jaunt in the other direction.

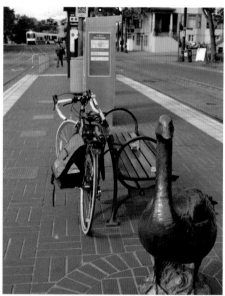

The downtown Portland area abounds with bronze statues.

Cedar Hills to Sylvan Hills

Please note: the profile for Ride 32 is depicted in 200ft vertical increments due to unusually high elevation.

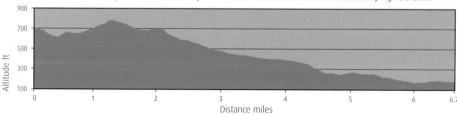

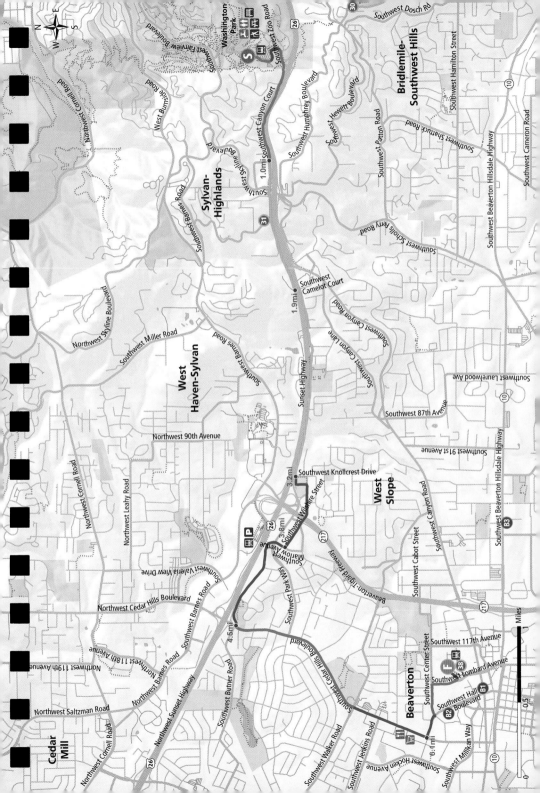

Hillsboro to Vernonia Ride 33

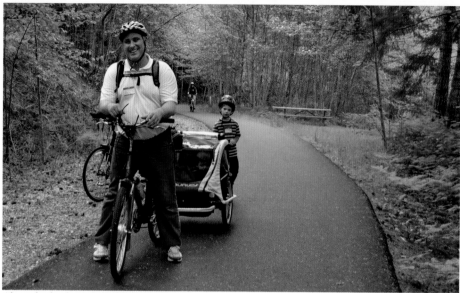

A happy family takes to the Banks-to-Vernonia Trail.

At a Glance
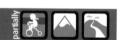

Distance 70.64 miles   **Elevation Gain** 5390'
Distance from Downtown Portland 18 miles

Terrain

Paved streets and multi-use pathway.

Traffic

Low-traffic roadways to the trailhead then smooth multi-use path to Vernonia. Expect to see pedestrians, horses, bicycles, skateboarders, and roller-bladers.

How to Get There

By car, take U.S. 26 west to Exit 62A NW Cornelius Pass Road S, right onto NE Cornell Road, right onto E Main Street; paid parking in garage or on-street parking.

By public transportation, take TriMet MAX Blue line train to the Hatfield Government Center MAX station.

Food and Drink

There is plenty of opportunity to fuel up in Hillsboro at the TriMet MAX station and at other retail establishments. Just before the trailhead the town of Banks offers another opportunity to replenish water and drinks, and again in Vernonia. At the trailhead, there are restrooms and drinking fountains, plus a bike shop that sells and rents bikes in addition to snacks and drinks.

Side Trip

The Banks-to-Vernonia Trail runs through Stub Stewart State Park which offers camping, cabins, and 20 miles of trails for hiking.

Links to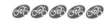

Where to Bike Rating

184 **Where to Bike** *Portland*

About...

The Banks-Vernonia Trail was awarded the 2011 Tourism and Hospitality Industry Award for its natural beauty and accessibility to Portland. The trail is a 21-mile linear state park along a former railroad line between Banks and Vernonia and has quickly become a favorite of local cyclists. Access the trail by beginning the trip with a 13-mile ride through beautiful farm and wine country beginning at the Hatfiled Government Center MAX station in downtown Hillsboro.

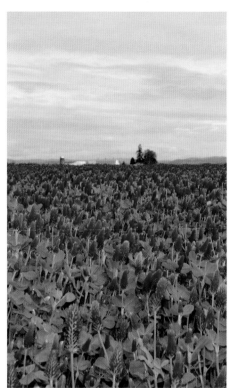

Spring flowers seem to go on forever along the road to Banks

The beginning of this trek brings cyclists through rolling farmland and vineyards. The road is rough but paved and crosses several railroad tracks between Hillsboro and Banks. Off in the distance are the foothills of the Coast Mountain Range. There is only one section of road that is along a busy street, Cornelius-Shefflin Road, but there is a wide bike lane along this section. The first part of the ride ends in the small town of Banks where the trailhead begins.

The Banks-to-Vernonia Trail has been in existence for some time, but there is one section that was only recently completed to bypass an old impassable railroad trestle. This section of the trail is called Tophill Trailhead. Be sure to take a moment to ride down the road a short ways to view the old wooden trestle that still bridges the road. The only notable climbing on the trail is in this section where switchbacks were built to provide an easier pathway to cross the street below.

Cyclists will enjoy crossing the other renovated 700-foot long, 80-foot high railroad trestle as well as the 13 wooden bridges that add to the splendor of the ride.

The trail bisects Stub Stewart State Park that offers year-round camping in cabins or tents. The park offers

miles of hiking trails and it is not uncommon to encounter horses along the trail. The park is named for L.L. "Stub" Stewart who served for 40 years on the State Parks and Recreation Advisory Committee and the Oregon Parks and Recreation Commission.

The town of Vernonia is directly across from Anderson Park and offers an opportunity to refuel. Anderson Park has a playground, restrooms and drinking fountains. The one mile loop around Lake Vernonia is just a short distance beyond the park on the right. This man-made lake is a favorite fishing spot.

On the return ride after leaving the Tophill Trailhead, cyclists may be surprised to find that they have a long descent where they need hardly pedal. The elevation rises slowly on the way out and offers a welcome glide into the Banks Trailhead before retracing the roads back through farm country to Hillsboro.

Ride Log

0.0 Take the Hillsboro TriMet MAX train to the Hatfield Government Center MAX station (end of the line).

0.03 Exit the station and travel west (left) on NW Main St.

0.16 Right on NW Cornell St.

0.6 Left on NW Garibaldi St.

0.9 Right on NW 10th Ave.

1.4 NW 10th turns into NW Padgett Rd at a bend in the road.

2.3 Turn right to stay on NW Padgett Rd.

3.7 Cross NW Hornecker Rd and dogleg left onto NW Leisy Rd. Railroad tracks ahead.

5.6 Left on NW Wren Rd. Railroad tracks ahead.

6.0 Right on NW Cornelius-Schefflin Rd.

8.9 Left on NW Roy Rd. Railroad tracks ahead.

10.9 Left on NW Wilkesboro Rd.

12.1 Right onto Rte 47; pass under the railroad bridge into the town of Banks.

12.1 Turn right to access the Banks-to-Vernonia Trailhead at the corner of NW Seller and NW Banks roads.

19.8 The trail has a slight incline until about the 20 mile mark just before the descent to the Tophill Trailhead; narrow and steep terrain is made easier to navigate by switchbacks in the trail on both sides of the road.

 P1 Lake Vernonia

33.1 Follow the trail without diverting until shortly after Anderson Park.

33.94 Turn right .84 miles after Anderson Park to follow the trail around Lake Vernonia which brings you back to the start in a one mile loop. Follow the trail without diverting to the Banks to Vernonia Trailhead.

54.94 Right out of the trailhead parking lot to the traffic light.

56.14 Left onto Rte 47.

58.14 Left onto NW Wilkesboro Rd.

61.04 Right onto NW Roy Rd. Railroad tracks ahead.

63.94 Right onto NW Cornelius-Schefflin Rd.

64.34 Left onto NW Wren Rd. Railroad tracks ahead.

67.24 Cross NW Hornecker Rd and dogleg right onto NW Leisy Rd.

68.64 Turn left to stay on NW Padgett Rd.

69.54 NW Padgett Rd turns into NW 10th at a bend in the road.

70.04 Right on NW 10th Ave.

70.48 Left on NW Garibaldi St.

70.61 Right on NW Cornell St.

70.64 Left on W Main St and return to Hatfield Government Center MAX station.

Hillsboro to Vernonia

Please note: the profile for Ride 33 is depicted in 200ft vertical increments due to unusually high elevation.

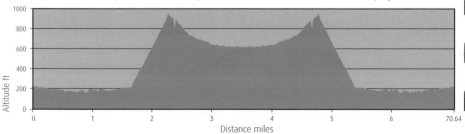

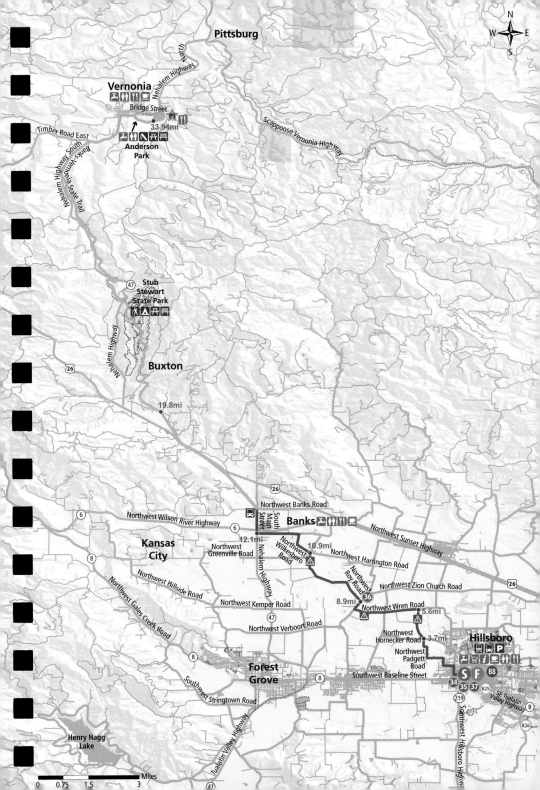

Pittsburg

Vernonia
Bridge Street
P1
33.94mi
Anderson
Park

Timber Road East
Nehalem Highway South
Banks-Vernonia State Trail
Nehalem Highway North
Scappoose Vernonia Highway

(47) Stub
Stewart
State Park

Nehalem Highway

Buxton

(26)

19.8mi

(6)

Northwest Wilson River Highway

Kansas
City

(6)

Northwest Banks Road
(26)
South
Main
Street
Banks

12.1mi
Northwest
Greenville Road
Northwest
Wilkesboro
Road
10.9mi
Northwest Harrington Road
Northwest Sunset Highway

Nehalem Highway

Northwest Kemper Road

(8)
Northwest Hillside Road

Northwest Gales Creek Road

(47)
Northwest Verboort Road

Northwest
Roy Road
(36)
8.9mi
Northwest Wren Road
5.6mi
Northwest Zion Church Road
(26)

Northwest
Hornecker Road
3.7mi
Hillsboro
P

Northwest
Padgett
Road

(8)

(8)

Forest
Grove

(8)
Southwest Baseline Street

S F
B8
(34)
(35)(37)

Southwest Stringtown Road

Henry Hagg
Lake

Tualatin Valley Highway

(47)

Southwest Hillsboro Highway
SE Tualatin
Valley Highway
(8)
(219)
K25
K26

Miles
0   0.75   1.5   3

N
W   E
S

Hillsboro Stroll

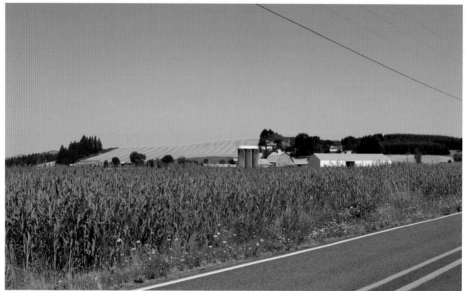

Farmland with rolling hills provides great scenery through the back roads and byways of Hillsboro and Forest Grove.

At a Glance

Distance 41.6 miles **Elevation Gain** 1790'
Distance from Downtown Portland 18.3 miles

Terrain

Rough roads, some shoulder-less. Root eruptions in places.

Traffic

Short section of urban traffic, then low-traffic roads.

How to Get There

By car, take 26 west to exit 69A to Route 217 south toward Beaverton/Tigard; take exit 2 onto OR-8/Canyon Road; right onto SW Canyon Road; road becomes TV Highway and then SE 10th Avenue; left onto E Main Street. On-street parking.

  By public transportation, take TriMet MAX Blue line train to Hillsboro; Hatfield Government Center MAX station is the last stop. By Bus, take #57 from the Beaverton Transit Center.

Food and Drink

At the TriMet MAX station there is both a deli and a hot dog stand. A short distance into town there are numerous restaurants and convenience stores.

Side Trip

Three vineyards – Plum Hill Vineyards, Patton Valley Vineyards, Montinore Estate – and one craft Sake bottler, Sake One.

Links to   37

Where to Bike Rating

About...

A stroll through Hillsboro would not be complete without riding by fields of wheat and corn, over rolling hills that pass by vineyards with ripening grapes hanging heavy on the vine. Add a loop around beautiful Hagg Lake and you have the recipe for this iconic rural Oregon bike ride. Much of the route out is flat, the ride back has some small rolling hills, but climbing the hills around Hagg Lake provides you with stunning views.

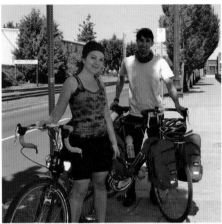

A weekend cycling adventure through wine country for this couple.

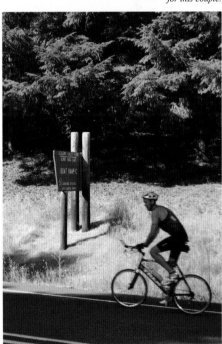

A lone cyclist begins the ascent to ride around Hagg Lake.

Beginning in Hillsboro center you'll have to endure the short ride along Route 8 west to Cornelius before turning off onto more rural roads that bring you out to farm country along a bike path and the turn off toward Hagg Lake. The ride becomes much quieter and riding single file along the shoulder-less road is no longer necessary. Riding on a sunny day, with the good conversation of fellow cyclists, and the smell of freshly harvested wheat fields is my favorite way to spend a Sunday morning. Life doesn't get much better...

If you plan well, you can bring an extra pannier or small trailer so that when you visit one (or more!) of the local vineyards along the route you can buy some wine for the picnic you'll want to have when you ride around Hagg Lake. My recommendation would be to ride about half way around the lake before stopping so you have an expansive view of the lake. There are several picnic areas, 15 miles of hiking trails, and the lake is fully stocked for those who enjoy fishing. Bird watching at one of the observation decks provides quiet relaxation before tackling the hills on the second half of the ride around the lake.

The return trip to Hillsboro Center brings you along rural roads through farm country. In the spring the clover fields bloom in stunning bursts of color, summer provides views of patchwork fields of grain, and in September the blackberry bushes are bursting with plump, ripe fruit that provide a great snack along the side of the road.

Ride Log

0.0 Begin at the Hillsboro Hatfield Government Center MAX station and ride west along OR 8, also known as E Baseline St. This becomes N Adair St and then Pacific Ave.

4.7 Left at Quince St onto Tualatin Valley Hwy (aka TV Hwy Route 47) and pick up the bike path.

9.8 Right onto SW Scoggins Valley Rd.

13.3 Left onto W Shore Dr, which is the first left upon entering Scoggins Valley State Park, toward Sain Creek and ride clockwise around Hagg Lake.

19.3 W Shore Dr becomes SW Scoggins Valley Rd at about the halfway point around the lake.

23.6 Exit the park via SW Scoggins Valley Rd.

27.0 Right onto Tualitin Valley Hwy Route 47 toward Gaston.

28.7 Left onto SW Gaston Rd, aka Main St.

29.6 Left at 4-way stop onto SW Springhill Rd.

32.5 Right onto SW Fern Hill Rd.

35.4 Right onto SW Geiger Rd.

36.2 Left onto SW Lafollett Rd.

37.2 Left onto SW Golf Course Rd which becomes S 10th Ave.

38.1 Right onto Baseline St, aka OR 8, after crossing the railroad tracks.

41.4 Left onto Adair St.

41.6 Return to Hillsboro Hatfield Government Center MAX station. End ride.

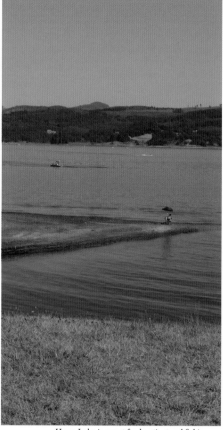

Hagg Lake is great for boating and fishing, or just enjoying the view.

Hillsboro Stroll

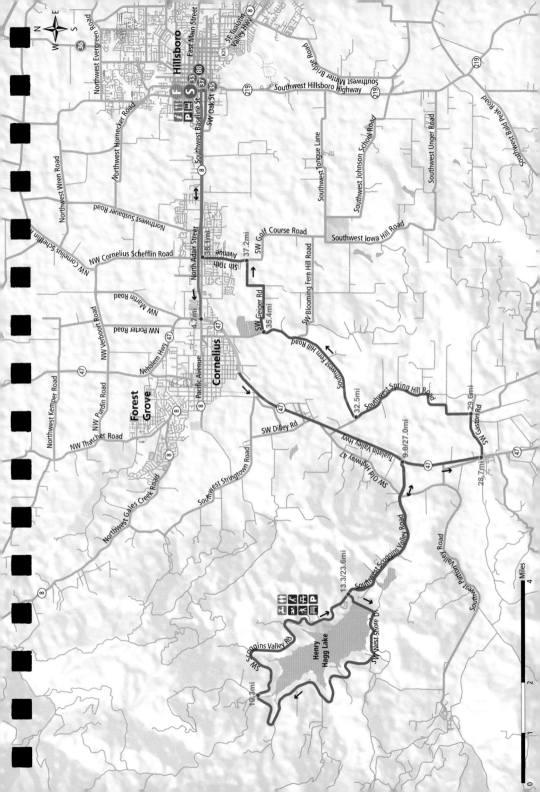

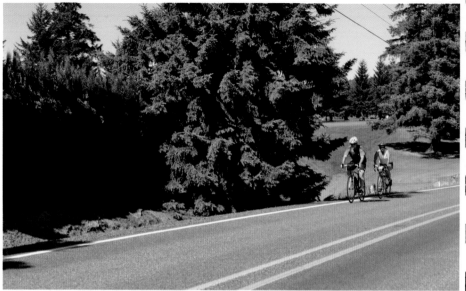

Challenging hills and breath-taking scenery keep this ride interesting at every turn.

At a Glance

Distance 21.6 miles   **Elevation Gain** 1423'
Distance from Downtown Portland 18.3 miles

Terrain

Paved roads of varying quality, many without shoulders and some with rough surfaces.

Traffic

Very low traffic beyond Hillsboro Center.

How to Get There

By car, take US 26 west to exit 69A to Highway 217 south toward Beaverton/Tigard; take exit 2 onto OR-8/ Canyon Road; right onto SW Canyon Road; road becomes TV Highway and then SE 10th Avenue; left onto E Main Street. Parking available in parking garage or on-street.

By public transportation, take TriMet MAX Blue line to Hillsboro; Hatfield Government Center station is the last stop. By bus, take #57 from the Beaverton Transit Center.

Food and Drink

There are numerous restaurants and convenience stores at the start and end of the ride, but once outside Hillsboro Center there is no food and drink available.

Side Trip

Shute Park is a great location for a picnic; two vineyards along the way offer tasting rooms; Rood Bridge Park has playgrounds and bike paths; two golf courses on this route are worth a return visit.

Links to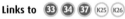

Where to Bike Rating

About...

Oregon sits at the same latitude as France which explains why the vineyards here produce some of the finest wines. Starting in Hillsboro center this ride quickly takes you into the countryside past two wineries with tasting rooms. The Jackson Bottom Wetlands preserve has helped to maintain the surrounding area as a lush rural farming community. In addition to the vineyards, the nurseries along this route produce a large variety of ornamental plants and trees that give the countryside wonderfully varying colors. A visual feast for the cyclist!

Just a short ride beyond Hillsboro Center is Jackson Bottom Wetlands. This 725 acre wildlife preserve offers quiet open waters, rolling meadows, and woods that are home to thousands of birds, beavers, deer, and otters. The preserve has a resource center that provides educational resources to school children, bird watchers, and researchers interested in wetlands and aquatic education.

Forest Hills Golf Course was built in 1927 and is one of the few remaining courses nestled in rolling foothills and beautiful farmland. The fairways are tree-lined, the greens well-manicured, and the bunkers are placed to provide sufficient challenge for all levels of golfers. Several of the golf holes provide views of Mount Hood, Mount St. Helens and Mount Adams.

Around the corner from "The Hills" is A Blooming Hill Vineyard & Winery which is located on a hillside of rich volcanic soil. The 480 foot elevation is protected by higher hills on three sides from harsh weather. These conditions help to warm the grapes and produce a very fine Pinot Noir.

At about the half-way point in the ride you will find Oak Knoll Winery. Established in 1970, this winery was the first in Washington County. With ancestors

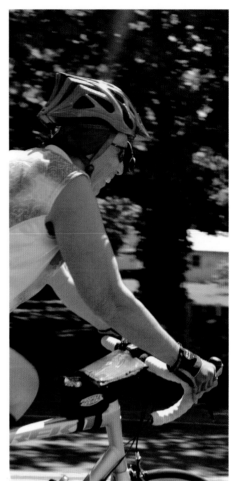

This rider is all smiles as she turns the corner and finds a welcome downhill ahead.

from the Bordeaux region of France, it is no wonder that this family-owned winery has produced outstanding Chardonnay, Pinot Gris, Pinot Noir, and Riesling wines.

On the return leg of the route is Meriwether National Golf Course which you will find on Rood Bridge Road. The course offers 27 regulation holes built along the Tualatin River and surrounded by farmland. The course provides a mix of open spaces, trees, ponds and indigenous birds and wildlife. Both Forest Hills and Meriwether National Golf Course offer memberships at reasonable rates.

West

Ride Log

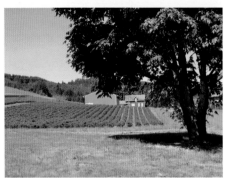

An idyllic farmhouse sitting on a hillside.

0.0 Begin at the Hillsboro Hatfield Government Center MAX station.

0.1 Left out of station to S First Ave; also Highway 219.

0.4 Right onto S First; Cross Walnut St and pick up bike lane. Watch for railroad tracks. You'll soon be out in the country. Narrow bike lane on two lane road but it's nice and flat. Go by Jackson Bottom Wetlands on left and cross Tualatin River. Road is a little rough in places.

2.8 Right onto S Tongue Ln. Through farmland you'll lose the bike lane, but traffic is light here.

5.7 Right onto SW Golf Course Rd directly across from the Forest Hills Golf Course.

6.0 Short way then left onto SW Blooming Fern Hill Rd; pass by Blooming Fern Hill Vineyard & Winery with tasting room. This is where the hills begin.

7.1 Left onto SW Hergbert Rd.

7.8 Left onto SW Nursery Rd; the road ends at a cemetery.

8.8 Right onto SW Iowa Hill Rd. At the top of the hill (quite a hill!) you'll be glad to know that your hills have not ended yet

10.0 Left onto SW Dober Rd and continue climbing. Every uphill is rewarded with a great downhill and this is no exception. Enjoy the farmland on both sides of the road as you come zooming down the hill.

11.2 Left onto SW Riedweg Rd; this road has a multitude of sharp turns and the pavement is rough with several hills.

13.4 Right onto SW Simpson Rd and cross over Highway 219.

15.4 Slight right onto SW Burkhalter Rd and go by the Oak Knoll Winery.

18.4 Left onto Rood Bridge Rd; you will be coming into more residential area. Pass by the Meriwether National Golf Course and the Rood Bridge Park.

18.6 Right at Hillsboro High School.

19.8 Left at traffic light is SE River Rd; there is a right turn lane, so bicycles need to move into the middle of the road and take a left with the traffic.

20.4 Left onto Tualatin Valley Hwy (TV Highway). This is a busy road, but there is a bike lane.

21.2 Left onto SE Walnut St; make a box turn at this busy, multi-lane road.

21.6 Right onto S First Ave, then left onto S. Washington St to return to the Hatfield Government Center MAX station. End ride

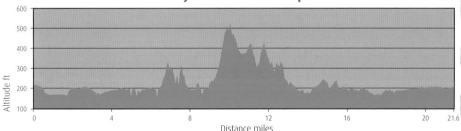

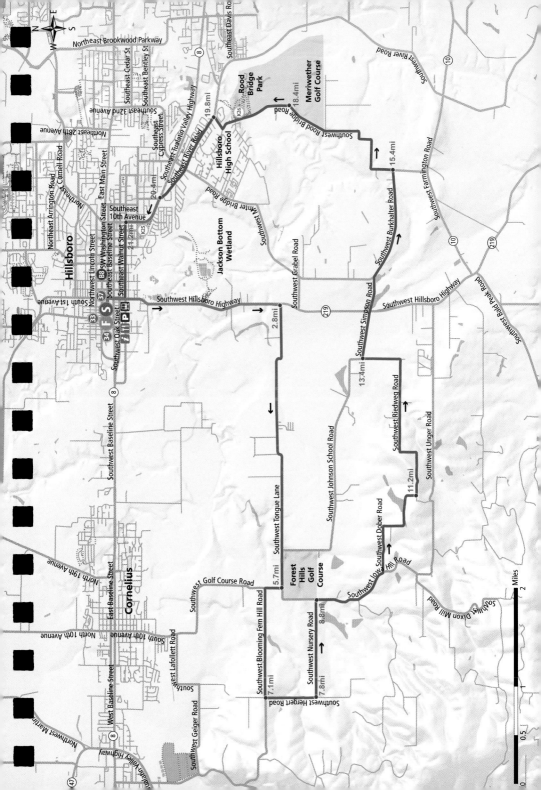

Hillsboro Farmlands

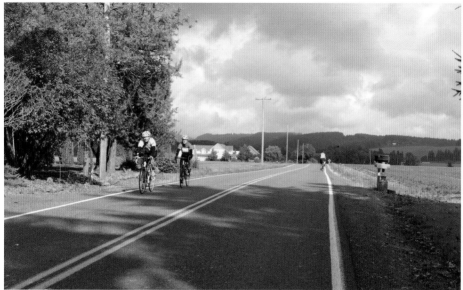

Rural roads are well paved and provide scenic vistas.

At a Glance

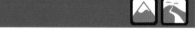

Distance 38.4 miles   **Elevation Gain** 1750'
Distance from Downtown Portland 14.7 miles

Terrain

Smooth, well-maintained streets in Hillsboro, some with bike lanes, then paved, narrow rural roads with narrow shoulders.

Traffic

Moderate traffic on urban streets in Hillsboro, then low-traffic rural roads.

How to Get There

By car, take U.S. Route 26 west and merge onto NW Cornelius Pass Road, turn right onto NE Cornell Road then left onto NE 231st Avenue and right onto NE Alder Street. On-street parking.

   By public transportation, take any red or blue line TriMet MAX train west to Orenco MAX station in Hillsboro.

Food and Drink

There are several small shops close by the Orenco TriMet MAX station to provide options for food and drink. About six miles from the end of the ride there is a restaurant on Helvetia Road. No public restrooms available.

Side Trip

Old Scotch Church, Helvetia Tavern, Jackson Bottom Wetlands.

Links to

Where to Bike Rating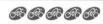

About...

This area of Hillsboro is a sensory delight of farmland, distant mountains, and golden wheat fields, not to mention the chickens, goats, and llamas you'll see along the way.

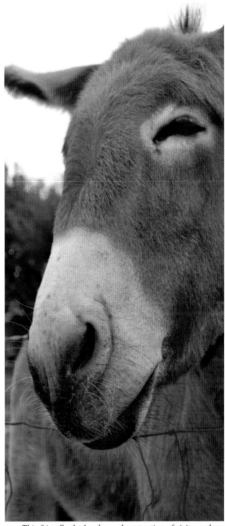

Leaving the Orenco MAX station in suburban Hillsboro you will ride for about five miles on wide multi-lane roads with bike lanes. The ride becomes distinctly more rural once you turn onto Jackson School Road and remains so for the next 28 miles. You'll pass the Old Scotch Church built in 1878 by Scottish Presbyterian immigrants. It's definitely worth stopping for a photo.

Most of the route is relatively flat until about the 25 mile mark. Then you'll find four hills. One on Mason Hill Road, one on Jackson Quarry Road, and the other two on Helvetia Road, the last of which is the highest peak. However, none of the hills is so challenging that you need to walk your bicycle with the highest peak at sub-500 feet. All provide opportunities for vista-viewing at their peaks.

The flat sections of the ride are along narrow paved rural roads with very low traffic. Though the shoulders are narrow, this is not a problem as you will not be competing for space with very many cars. You may encounter a horse or two, however. If you do this ride during the summer, you will pass by farms of golden waves of wheat and the occasional vineyard.

A short diversion up Bishop Road will bring you to a llama farm. This road is unpaved and a bit steep but worth the side trip to see the llamas up close. The return ride along Helvetia Road brings you to a delightful and popular restaurant with a front deck designed for tired and thirsty cyclists to enjoy refueling. It sits across from a farm with goats and donkeys that enjoy the attention of visitors.

This friendly donkey loves the attention of visitors along Helvetia Road.

Turning onto NW Jacobson Road you return to suburbia quickly and ride through a residential neighborhood. Pick up the bike/pedestrian trail at Rock Creek Park to avoid the heavily traveled NW 185th Avenue. The only sections of the ride that have heavy traffic are the first and last mile.

West

Ride Log

0.0 Begin at the corner of NE Orenco Station Parkway and NE Campus Court.

0.2 Right onto NE Cornell Rd.

0.5 Left onto NW 229th Ave.

1.7 Left onto NW Evergreen Parkway.

4.9 Right onto NW Jackson School Rd.

6.5 Left onto NW Scotch Church Rd.

8.2 Cross NW Glencoe Rd to access NW Zion Church Rd which becomes NW Cornelius-Schefflin Rd.

10.6 Right onto NW Roy Rd.

14.3 Right onto NW Mountaindale Rd.

14.6 Left onto NW Wilkesboro Mountain Rd.

15.0 Right onto NW Mountaindale Rd.

18.7 Road turns left.

19.9 Left onto NW North Ave.

20.9 Left onto NW Shadybrook Rd.

23.4 Right onto NW Jackson School Rd.

24.6 Left onto NW Mason Hill Rd.

25.4 Right onto NE Jackson Quarry Rd.

27.4 Left onto NW Helvetia Rd.

28.6 Left onto NW Bishop Rd; to visit the Llama farm reverse then left onto NW Helvetia Rd.

29.8 Helvetia Tavern.

32.1 Left onto NW Jacobson Rd.

33.6 Right onto NW Cornelius Pass Rd.

33.8 Left onto NW Rock Creek Blvd.

35.1 Right onto bike path through Rock Creek Park.

35.4 Right on NW Evergreen Parkway.

36.6 Left onto NW 229th Ave.

37.9 Right onto NE Cornell Rd.

38.1 Left onto NE Orenco Station Parkway.

38.4 Left onto NE Campus Court. End ride.

 P1 Old Scotch Church
P2 Llama Farm

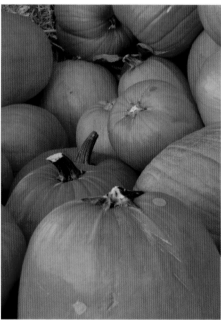

Autumn is colorful and the harvest abundant.

Hillsboro Farmlands

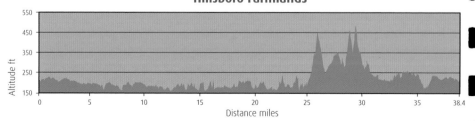

Altitude ft / Distance miles

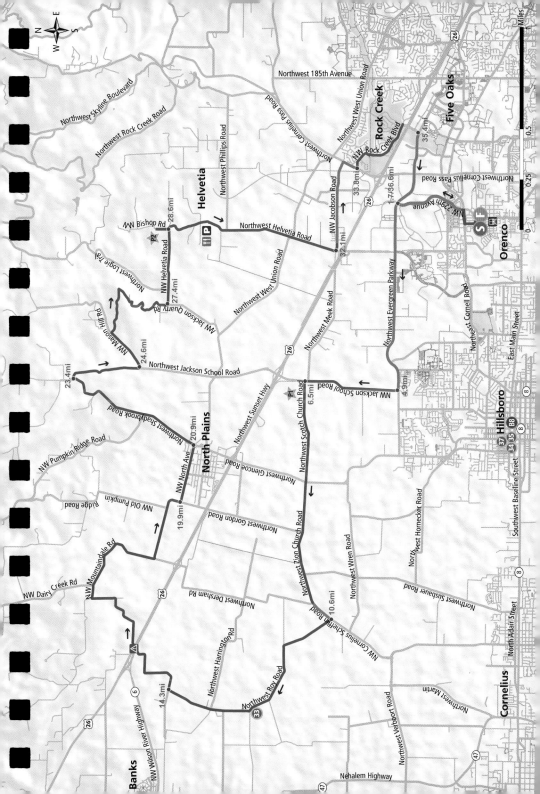

South

Variety is the spice of life and these rides offer plenty of flavors for your riding pleasure. Heading south to historic Champoeg State Park you will immerse yourself in the very beginnings of Oregon's history. The Clackamas River ride brings you up close to the days of the Conestoga wagons that were used on the Oregon Trail when this area was first settled. Bringing you full circle to modern day are two rides that highlight Portland neighborhoods and wine country agri-business.

Champoeg State Park is located at the southern-most point of the rides contained in this book. Many cyclists mount their bike on a car and then cycle around the area when they arrive. My recommendation is to be confident that you can make the trip on your bicycle by following the route designed here and still enjoy cycling the surrounding areas once you arrive. The history of the area is well worth the visit.

On another day you may wish to acquaint yourself with the history of the Oregon Trail by riding around the Clackamas River to gain an understanding of the challenges that must have faced the early settlers. On a hot summer day you may even be tempted to put your bike down and dip your toes in the river where you are sure to find lots of people floating along with the current.

How can anyone visit this area and not visit wine country? Not too far away are plenty of small farms producing a few bottles of wine from their backyard vineyards. They would be glad to share a taste with you and perhaps sell you a bottle or two. Panniers would be a good idea if you plan on stopping.

Circling back to town you can explore one of the residential neighborhoods in Southeast Portland where there are beautiful parks, lovely homes, and lots of fellow cyclists. Consider the rides in this section as a way to connect the early days of Oregon to today and make your own mark on history with a memorable day of exploration and learning.

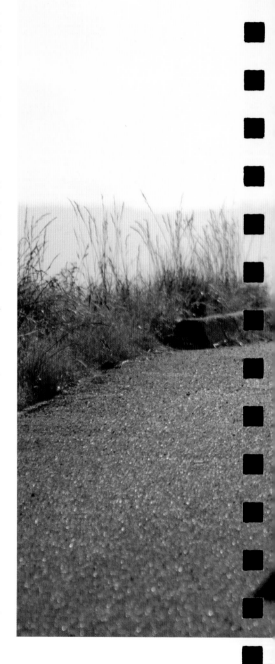

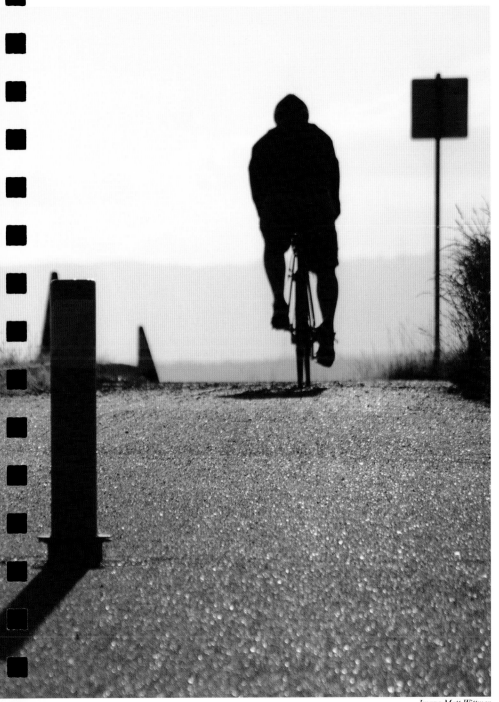

Image Matt Wittmer

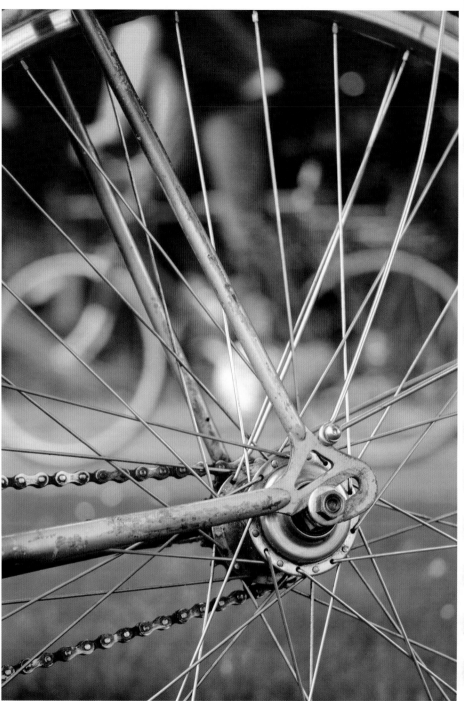

Image Matt Wittmer

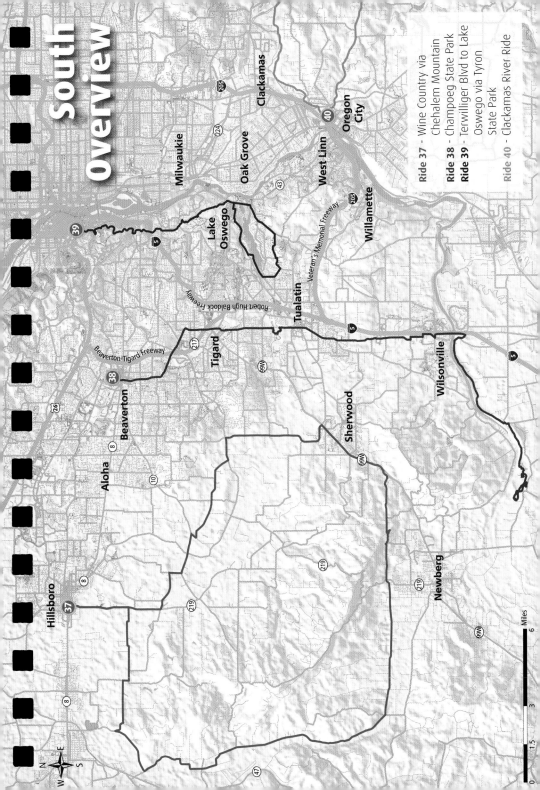

Ride 37 - Wine Country via Chehalem Mountain

Ride 38 - Champoeg State Park

Ride 39 - Terwilliger Blvd to Lake Oswego via Tyron State Park

Ride 40 - Clackamas River Ride

Clackamas

Milwaukie

Oak Grove

West Linn

Oregon City

Willamette

Lake Oswego

Veteran's Memorial Freeway

Robert Hugh Baldock Freeway

Tualatin

Tigard

Beaverton-Tigard Freeway

Beaverton

Aloha

Sherwood

Wilsonville

Hillsboro

Newberg

Miles

0   1.5   3   6

N
W   E
S

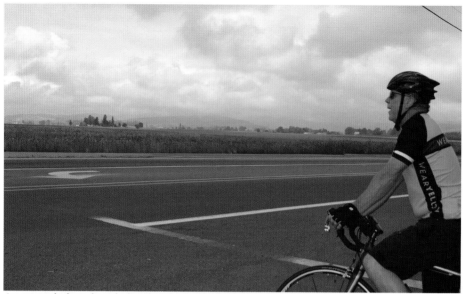

At a crossroads, this cyclist embarks on his ride through rural Hillsboro.

At a Glance

Distance 52.0 miles   **Elevation Gain** 3950'
Distance from Downtown Portland 18.3 miles

Terrain

Paved roads with varying quality from well-maintained to rough pavement. Some rural two-lane roads are narrow; others are multi-lane urban streets.

Traffic

Moderate traffic on urban streets in Hillsboro, then low-traffic rural roads.

How to Get There

By car, take U.S. Route 26 west to exit 69A to Highway 217 south toward Beaverton/Tigard; take exit 2 onto OR-8/Canyon Road; right onto SW Canyon Road; road becomes TV Highway and then SE 10th Avenue; left onto E Main Street. Parking on-steet.

By public transportation, take the TriMet Blue line to Hillsboro. Hatfield Government Center station

is the last stop. By bus, take #57 from the Beaverton Transit Center.

Food and Drink

At the MAX station in Hillsboro there is both a deli and a hot dog stand. A short distance into town there are numerous restaurants and convenience stores.

Side Trip

Tualatin River National Wildlife Refuge, Jackson Bottom Wetlands, and Forest Hills Golf Course.

Links to 33 34 35

Where to Bike Rating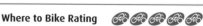

About...

The Willamette Valley is world renowned for its wine and produces some of the best Pinot noir in the world. Sitting on the same latitude as the Burgundy and Alsace regions of France, the conditions are excellent for vineyard grapes. Chehalem Mountain is one of six appellations in the Willamette Valley wine country which is home to two thirds of Oregon's wineries. This route is dotted with more than a dozen small wineries and tasting rooms.

Downtown Hillsboro, where this ride begins, gives way quickly to two-lane rural roads that circle around wine country. The countryside is abundant with vineyards and small make-shift signs urge passersby to visit the local tasting rooms. Many of the vineyards are referred to as boutique wineries because of their small production. A few boast a major annual production. Visiting the smaller wineries will put you in touch with wine artisans who craft wines for local and personal palates. Most have tasting rooms where you can sip the local offerings and chat with the vineyard owners.

After leaving SW Roy Rogers Road, you will ride approximately three miles along the Pacific Highway, a busy, multi-lane road with a bike lane before taking a right onto SW Bell Road that will bring you up Chehalem Mountain. The steep hill masks the second ascent necessary before reaching the summit, and is the highest peak on the ride. A second, smaller hill waits at mile 44 with a sub-400 foot peak but a 13 percent grade.

After leaving Chehalem Mountain behind, the ride becomes much flatter and more serene as you pass quiet farm fields. Turning onto SW Hillsboro Highway brings you the two miles back to downtown Hillsboro. This road is moderately traveled and the traffic speed

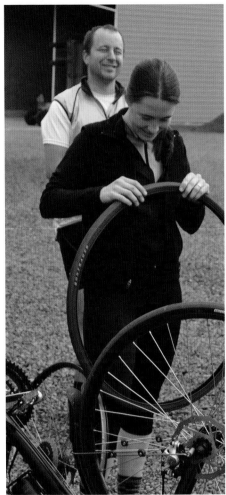

Even a flat tire cannot dampen the spirits of these intrepid cyclists.

much faster. There is a shoulder that accommodates bicycles, however.

If you are planning to do some wine tasting along the way be sure to bring food with you so that your travel will not pose a risk to yourself and others on the road. In Oregon bicycles are vehicles and subject to the same laws as motor vehicles. Cyclists can be arrested for driving under the influence. To make this ride memorable in the best possible way, plan to sip small quantities, eat, and take your time.

Ride Log

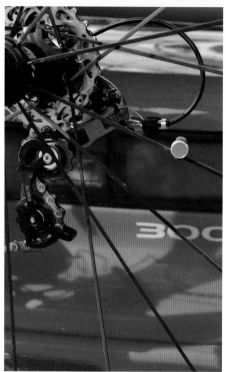

Beloved vehicles perfectly matched.

0.0 Begin at the Hillsboro Government Center TriMet MAX station; left along SW Washington St.

0.1 Right onto S First Ave (also known as SW Hillsboro Hwy).

4.1 Left onto SW Burkhalter Rd.

5.6 Right onto SW Rood Bridge Rd.

6.1 Left onto SW Farmington Rd.

7.7 Right onto SW Tile Flat Rd.

11.6 Left onto SW Scholls Ferry Rd.

12.5 Right onto SW Roy Rodgers Rd.

17.0 Right onto SW Pacific Hwy.

20.0 Right onto SW Bell Rd (becomes NE Bell Rd).

25.0 Left onto NE North Valley Rd.

34.2 Cross NE Albertson Rd to continue on NE Spring Hill Rd (becomes SW Spring Hill Rd).

41.7 Right onto SW Fern Hill Rd.

43.8 Right onto SW Blooming Fern Hill Rd.

46.0 Right onto SW Golf Course Rd.

46.3 Left onto SW Tongue Ln.

49.3 Left onto SW Hillsboro Hwy.

51.9 Left onto SE Washington St.

52.0 Right into the Hillsboro Government Center Tri-Met MAX station. End ride.

Wine Country via Chehalem Mountain

Please note: the profile for Ride 37 is depicted in 200ft vertical increments due to unusually high elevation.

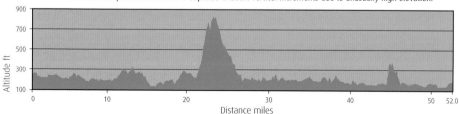

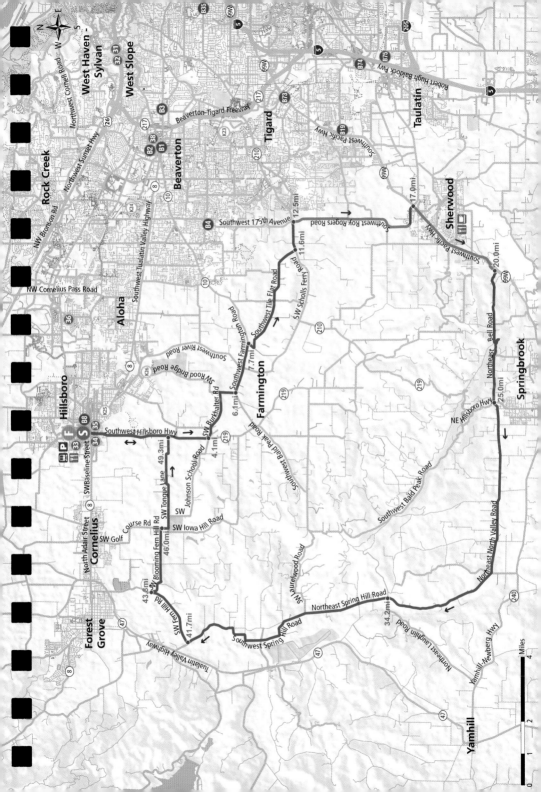

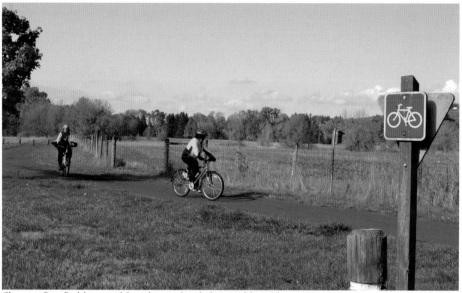

Champoeg State Park has many bike paths to explore the history of the rural community.

At a Glance

Distance 52.9 miles   **Elevation Gain** 2416′

Distance from Downtown Portland 7.2 miles

Terrain

Paved roads with bike lanes or wide shoulders, and some rough bike paths in Champoeg State Park.

Traffic

Moderate traffic on suburban streets in Beaverton, Route I-5 crossing is multi-lane highway traffic, and finally low-traffic rural roads.

How to Get There

By car, take US 26 west to exit 71A to merge onto SW Canyon Road, turn right onto SW Lombard Avenue to Beaverton Transit Center Tri-Met MAX station. No parking at Beaverton TC. On-street parking within a half mile from the station. Because of the inconvenient parking situation, it is recommended to take public transportation.

By public transportation, take the Red or Blue Tri-Met MAX line west to the Beaverton Transit Center MAX station. Buses #58 and #54 from downtown Portland and the WES commuter rail from Wilsonville.

Food and Drink

At the Beaverton MAX station there is a small snack shack. Along the route there are numerous opportunities for food and drink in Beaverton, Tigard, Tualatin, and Wilsonville.

Side Trip

Cook Park, Durham City Park, Butterfly Garden, and the Butteville General Store.

Links to (32) (K23)

Where to Bike Rating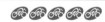

About...

Champoeg State Park is a cycling destination because of the wonderful bike paths through and around the park. To drive to the park is to miss some of the joy of the journey however. The towns of Beaverton, Tigard, Tualatin, and Wilsonville have made major strides in constructing bike-friendly streets. On the way, you'll ride through Cook Park in Tualatin before taking Route I-5 across the Tualatin River, a thrilling experience to be sure.

Travelling through Beaverton, Tigard, Tualatin, and Wilsonville on the way to Butteville is quite comfortable with bike lanes all along the way. There are ample opportunities to stop and rest or refuel as you find necessary. The ride will take you on suburban roads and through two parks – Tualatin Community Park where you will find a butterfly garden – before you reach Champoeg State Park.

Champoeg State Park is a wonderful mix of history, nature and recreation. There is much to do beyond bicycling, but cycling is definitely one of the best ways to enjoy all that the park offers. The historic buildings and Pioneer Mothers Log Cabin Museum take you back in time to the days of the Wild West, which you will discover is a short 150 or so years in the past. There are nature walks, bike tours, and programs to learn about how the settlers lived in this area on the south bank of scenic Willamette River.

One of the biggest thrills of the ride, however, is traversing the Tualatin River via I-5. There being no other bridge, the only way to cross the river is via the I-5 highway. Pick up the on-ramp in Wilsonville and ride one exit south. I am sure that in an automobile this is a very fast trip, but on a bicycle with vehicles speeding past at 60 miles per hour, it is both nerve-wracking and thrilling in equal measure. And since this is an out-and-back ride, you'll get to experience the thrill twice.

One more must along this ride is a visit to the Historical Butteville Store, the oldest operating store in the state, founded in 1863. Riding through this community and state park is to truly connect with the earliest days of Oregon history.

Ride Log

0.0 Begin at Beaverton Transit Center TriMet MAX station, right (west) on SW Lombard St.

0.02 Left onto SW Center St.

0.5 Left onto SW Hall Blvd.

0.6 SW Hall Blvd splits; continue straight on SW Watson Ave.

1.5 SW Watson Ave rejoins SW Hall Blvd; continue on SW Hall Blvd.

7.9 Cross SW Durham Rd onto SW 85th Ave; at end of road, continue into Cook Park.

9.1 Right onto bike/pedestrian path to continue into Tualatin Community Park.

9.6 Exit park onto SW Tualatin Rd which becomes SW Boones Ferry Rd after crossing SW Tualatin-Sherwood Rd.

13.2 Jog right at SW Commerce Court onto SW 95th Ave.

14.6 Left onto Boeckman Rd.

14.7 Right onto Boberg Rd.

15.2 Left onto SW Barber St.

15.3 Right onto Wilsonville Frontage Rd (also known as SW Boones Ferry Rd).

15.9 Left onto SW Wilsonville Rd.

16.0 Right onto Route I-5 entrance ramp (remain on I-5 one exit) and cross Tualatin River.

17.2 Exit I-5 and take right onto NE Miley Rd.

17.4 Right onto NE Butteville Rd (also known as First St NE).

22.0 Left onto Second St NE (also known as Butteville Rd NE).

South

Ride Log

22.2 Right onto Schuler Rd NE to access the bike entrance to Champoeg State Park.

24.3 At end of path take a right to continue into the park.

24.5 Right into parking lot at Townsite Trail; circle and exit onto bike path.

24.9 Right onto bike path to continue into the park.

25.5 Right onto bike/pedestrian path to far end.

26.4 Right to continue on bike/pedestrian path to return to starting point.

27.3 Right on path to cross road and ascend hill to museum.

28.4 Left to exit bike/pedestrian path to exit park.

30.0 Access SE Schuler Rd NE.

30.5 Left onto Butteville Rd NE (also known as Second St NE).

30.7 Left at Butteville General Store onto NE Butteville Rd (also known as First St NE). Right to remain on Butteville Rd NE.

35.3 Left onto NE Miley Rd.

35.6 Left onto I-5 one exit.

36.9 Left onto SW Wilsonville Rd at the end of the exit ramp.

37.1 Right onto SW Boones Ferry Rd.

37.6 Left onto SW Barber St.

37.7 Right onto Boberg Rd.

38.2 Left onto Boeckman Rd.

38.3 Right onto SW 95th Ave.

39.8 Right at SW Commerce Court and then left onto SW Boones Ferry Rd.

43.3 Enter Tualatin Community Park

43.9 Left at end of bike path into Cook Park.

44.6 Exit Cook Park onto SW 85th Ave.

45.1 Cross SW Durham Rd onto SW Hall Blvd.

52.5 Right onto SW Center St.

52.7 Right onto SW Lombard St.

52.9 Left into Beaverton Transit Center TriMet MAX station. End ride.

 P1 Cook Park
P2 Champoeg State Park

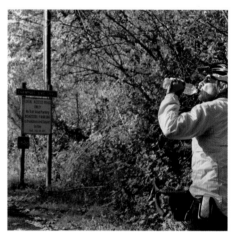

At the entrance to the park, this cyclist takes a break before exploring all that Champoeg offers.

Champoeg State Park

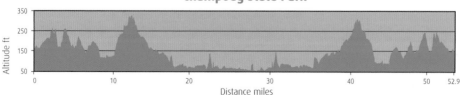

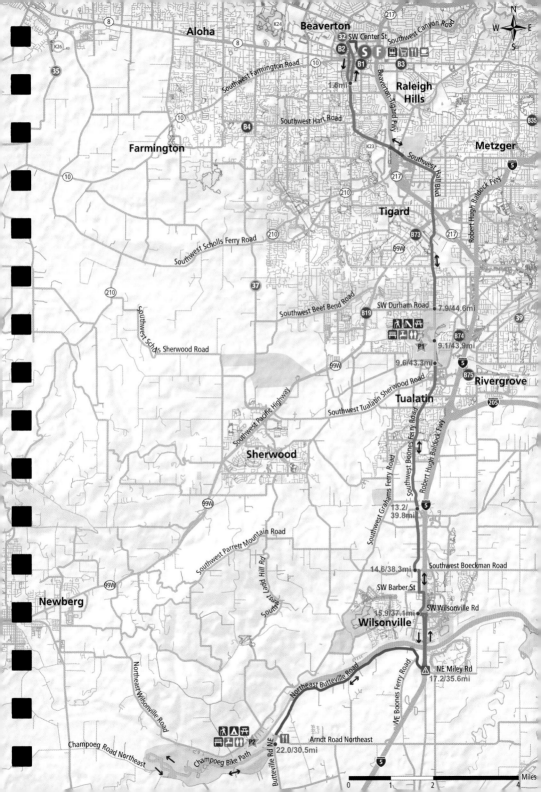

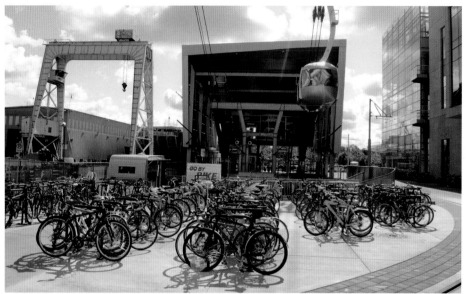

Consider Portland's Aerial Tram a fitting beginning, or end, to today's journey.   Image Matt Wittmer

At a Glance

Distance 25.0 miles   **Elevation Gain** 2760'
Distance from Downtown Portland 0.5 miles

Terrain

Smooth roadways. Avoid the reflectors embedded along the edge of the road riding down Iron Mountain Road.

Traffic

Bike lanes from downtown Portland through urban traffic, bike paths through Tryon Creek State Park, and low-traffic roads around the lake.

How to Get There

By car, park anywhere downtown Portland near the South Park blocks.

   By public transportation, buses numbered 6, 38, 43, 58, 68, and 96 to the South Park blocks stop at #1108 on SW Columbia Street.

Food and Drink

Food and drink are abundantly available downtown before beginning the ride and again in the town center of Lake Oswego. There are restrooms in Tryon Creek State Park.

Side Trip

Saturday farmers' market on the campus of Portland State University; Pioneer Square, aka Portland's Living Room; the Waterfront; Campbell's Native Garden in Lake Oswego.

Links to 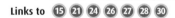 15 21 24 26 27 28 30

Where to Bike Rating

About...

Riding over Terwilliger Boulevard from downtown Portland will provide a wonderful vista of three bridges over the Willamette River. After crossing a couple of busy intersections picturesque downtown Lake Oswego awaits on the other side of the densely-forested Tryon Creek State Park. This ride abounds with hills that are worth the effort in order to get glimpses through the trees of downtown Portland and scenic Lake Oswego.

One of my favorite routes to exit the downtown Portland is via Terwilliger Boulevard that ascends Marquam Hill traveling south. You'll pass by the esteemed Oregon Health and Science University and under the aerial tram that brings people from the river up the side of the hill to the upper OHSU campus. After crossing SW Barbur Boulevard you'll ride through the Burlingame neighborhood via a bike lane to the corner of SW Taylors Ferry Road where Tryon Creek State Park begins. Riding through this linear park it is hard to imagine that you are traveling parallel to busy Terwilliger Boulevard. The bike/pedestrian path meanders through the cool, dark forest. On the hot summer day of our ride there were lots of joggers and walkers enjoying the cool shade of this park that is tucked away between Portland and Lake Oswego.

The bike path brings you to the road that travels through downtown Lake Oswego. I so enjoy riding into this adorable downtown with the hanging flower baskets and sidewalk cafés, but I suggest that cyclists take care on this narrow main street.

The ride around the lake takes you through lovely neighborhoods along streets that front the lake. The architecture of the stately homes and manicured gardens

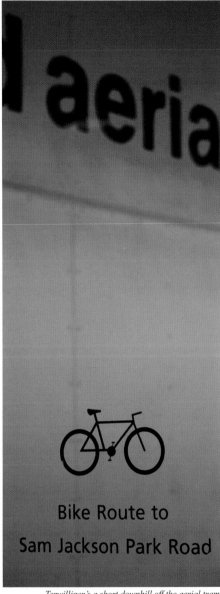

Terwilliger's a short downhill off the aerial tram.
Image Matt Wittmer

are worth taking a little extra time to slow down and enjoy. Along Iron Mountain Road we were startled as a doe leapt out in front of our bikes and darted across the road into the woods on the other side.

South

Ride Log

 P1 Lake Oswego
P2 Tryon Creek State Park

0.0 Begin at the corner of SW Columbia St and Broadway riding south up the hill.

0.6 Right onto SW Sixth Ave which becomes SW Terwilliger Blvd at SW Sheridan St.

1.0 Left at the traffic light to continue on SW Terwilliger Blvd.

5.6 Right at the traffic light where SW Taylors Ferry Rd joins SW Terwilliger Blvd and enter Tyron Creek State Park bike/pedestrian path.

8.3 Right onto N State St as you exit Tyron Creek State Park.

9.2 Right onto McVey Ave which becomes Stafford Rd at South Shore Blvd.

10.8 Right onto SW Overlook Dr.

11.8 Left onto Westview Rd then a right onto Royce Rd.

12.3 Right onto Bryant Rd.

13.2 Right onto Lakeview Blvd.

14.4 Right onto Iron Mountain Blvd.

15.9 Right onto Chandler Rd.

16.0 Right onto SW A Ave.

16.4 Left onto Fourth Ave.

16.5 Right onto SW B Ave.

16.7 Left onto N State St.

17.0 Left onto SW Terwilliger Blvd.

24.4 Straight through the traffic light onto SW Sixth Ave.

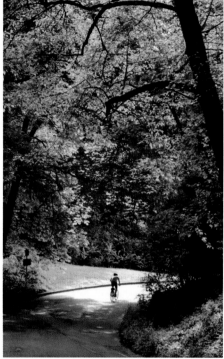
Come climbers, come all.   Image Matt Wittmer

24.9 Left onto SW Harrison St into the Portland State University campus.

25.0 Park your bike and enjoy Saturday farmers' market three blocks north of SW Columbia St. End ride.

Terwilliger Blvd to Lake Oswego via Tryon Creek State Park

Please note: the profile for Ride 39 is depicted in 200ft vertical increments due to unusually high elevation.

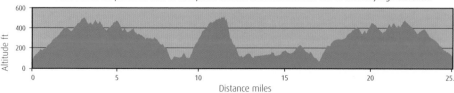

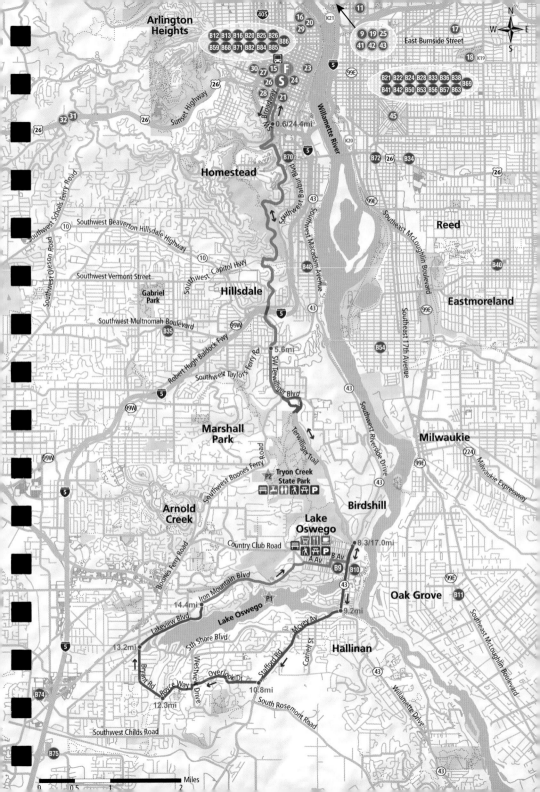

Clackamas River Ride

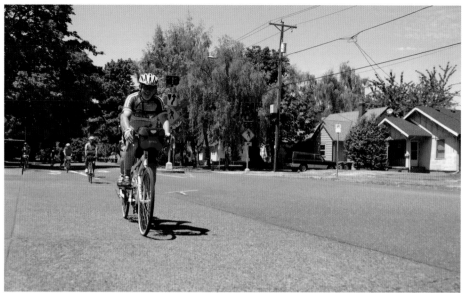

A happy cyclist!

At a Glance

Distance 25.0 miles **Elevation Gain** 1700'
Distance from Downtown Portland 14.6 miles

Terrain

Smooth, well-maintained streets, some narrow with no shoulder or bike lane.

Traffic

Narrow rural roads; some roads a little rough.

How to Get There

By car, take I-205 S/OR-213 S/OR-224 S toward Oregon City/Estacada; exit 10 for State 213 S toward Oregon City/Molalla; right onto OR-213 S/State 213 S/Washington Street; first right onto Washington Street. Parking available at the End of the Trail Interpretive Center on right.

By **public transportation**, take Bus #33 toward Clackamas Community College; disembark at Oregon City Transit Center, stop #97045.

Food and Drink

There are restrooms and drinking fountains at the End of the Trail Interpretive Center during posted hours.

Side Trip

Visit historic Oregon City and the End of the Trail Interpretive Center.

Where to Bike Rating

About...

In the spring the Clackamas River is swollen with the snow melt from Mount Hood, but in late summer it calms down to a slower pace that suits recreationists who enjoy both fishing and tubing. This route through quiet farms in rural Oregon City is a favorite of cyclists for its low-traffic roads, beautiful scenery, and challenging hills.

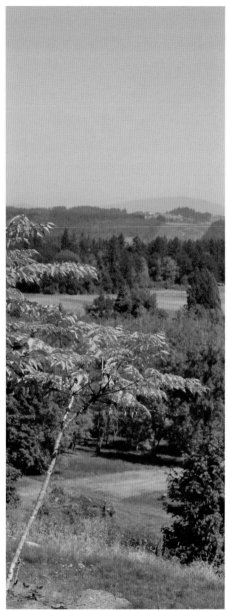

Clackamas River Drive parallels the Clackamas River as it weaves up and down alongside the occasional house. As you ride along you can peek through the trees to get a glimpse of the river rushing over boulders and around sand bars. The road will have some hills and some blind corners, but the motor vehicle traffic is light and you can ride in the roadway without too much concern.

It is important not to miss the turn off onto S Bakers Ferry Road because S Springwater Road is narrow and more heavily travelled. Bakers Ferry will bring you along beautiful horse farms. On the day of our ride, the fields were tall with spinach, corn, and other produce ready to be harvested.

When you turn onto S Eaden Road get ready for the most challenging hills on the ride. While steep, they are in a stair step pattern providing you with brief relief between climbs. The view from the top of the hill makes the effort worthwhile. Snow-capped even in summer, Mount Hood stands in the distance making this ride one to plan for a clear day.

Fischers Mill Road provides the awaited descent from the Eaden Road climb. When you turn the corner onto Redland Road you'll be coming back into a more densely populated area, but by no means does it qualify as "suburban" as you'll still be riding through an area

Scene from the highest peak of Clackamas River Ride.

of horse farms and nurseries. Return to the End of the Trail Interpretive Center where the Oregon Trail – and your ride – ends.

Ride Log

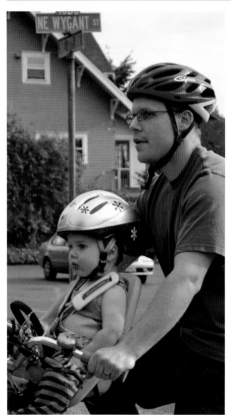

Sitting proudly on Dad's bike.

 P1 Oregon Interpretive Center

0.0 Begin at the parking lot of the End of the Trail Interpretive Center; right onto Washington St.

0.7 Cross Cascade Hwy onto Clackamas River Dr.

6.4 Clackamas River Dr becomes S Springwater Rd.

8.0 Right onto S Bakers Ferry Rd also known as Eagle Creek Rd.

10.8 S Bakers Ferry Rd becomes Harding Mill Rd.

11.0 Right onto S Eaden Rd.

15.2 Right onto S Springwater Rd then immediate left onto S Fischers Mill Rd.

19.2 Right onto S Redland Rd.

24.3 Left onto S Holcomb Blvd.

24.8 Right onto Washington St.

25.0 Return to parking lot of the End of the Trail Interpretive Center. End ride.

Clackamas River Ride

Please note: the profile for Ride 40 is depicted in 200ft vertical increments due to unusually high elevation.

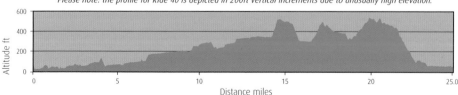

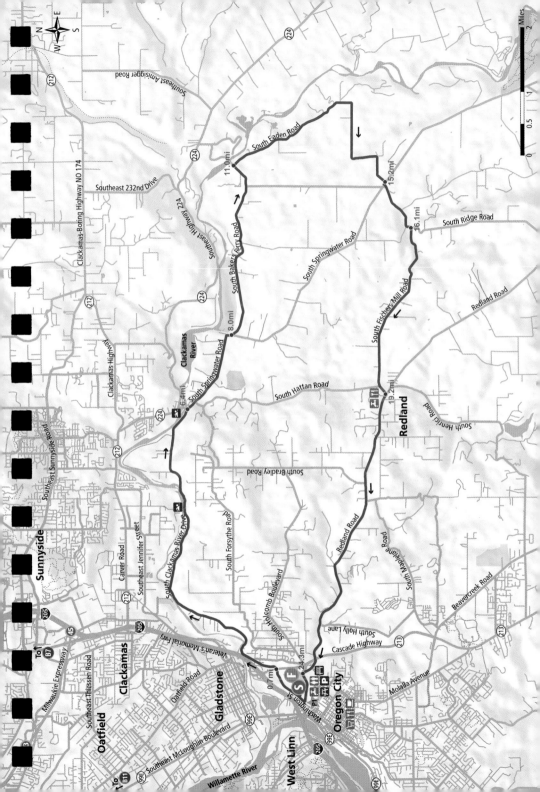

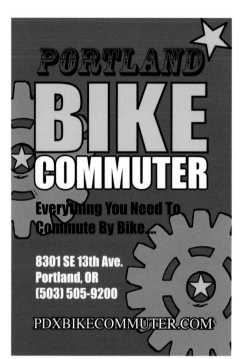
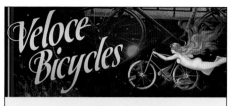
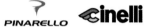
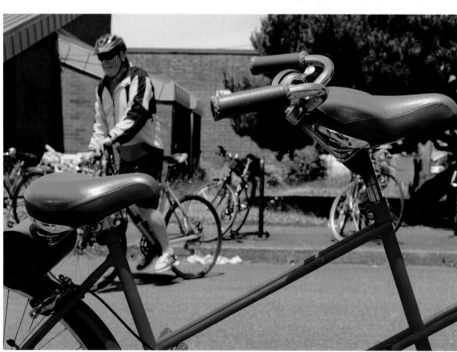

Images Matt Wittmer

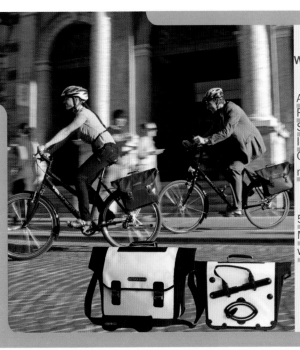
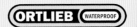
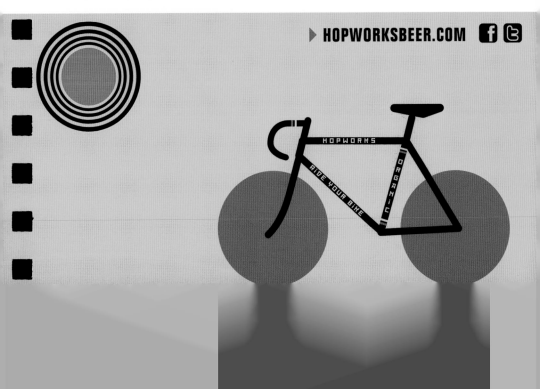

East

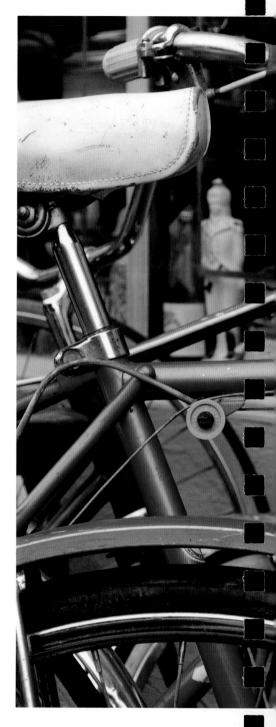

S ome of the most dramatic views and geologic history of this region are found in the Columbia River Gorge. Visiting this area would not be complete without a ride through the Gorge to Multnomah Falls. Equally enjoyable are the other rides in this section that tour the major bike paths east of the city and one that even brings you to a well-known flour miller.

The Columbia River has carved out amazing geologic patterns and in so doing created the Columbia River Gorge. The rock formations are amazing. Visitors will be hard-pressed to decide which is the most impressive – the expansive views of the gorge, the incredible waterfalls, or the lush green forests that surround you. There is no need to decide – just enjoy the ride. Also of interest to those who wish to explore the local landscape is the ride to two of the three volcanoes located within the city limits of Portland.

Closer to downtown Portland is Tryon State Park where you can explore the park and then ride around Lake Oswego. More residential than rural this ride brings you through the park with miles of biking and hiking trails before you begin your spin around the beautiful lake. This is a great ride for a day when you want to explore quaint downtown Lake Oswego and or have a picnic in one of the many parks. If staying on bike paths is more to your taste you can explore the entire length of the Route I-205 bike path or take the East Portland loop that will let you explore some of the early bike paths constructed east of the city.

If you are interested in the perfect destination for both a great lunch and a shopping trip, don't overlook Ride 43 to Bob's Red Mill. The mill is a great destination with its cafeteria-style restaurant and outdoor seating, making this a terrific group ride for family and friends.

This chapter will take you from close to downtown to the outskirts of Portland and closer to the geologic history of the region.

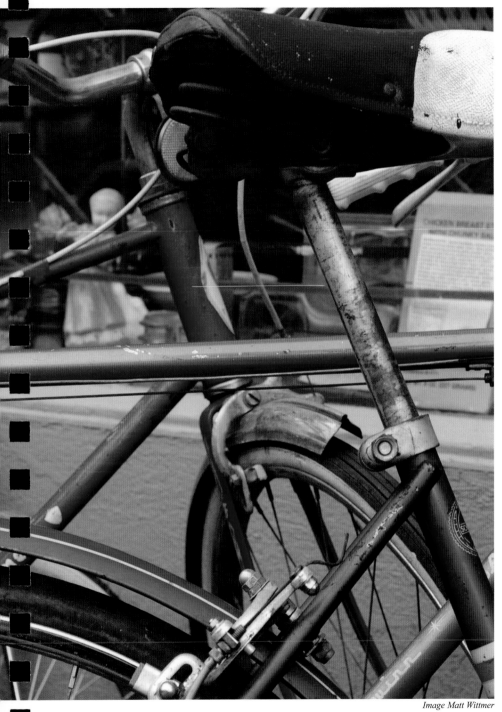

Image Matt Wittmer

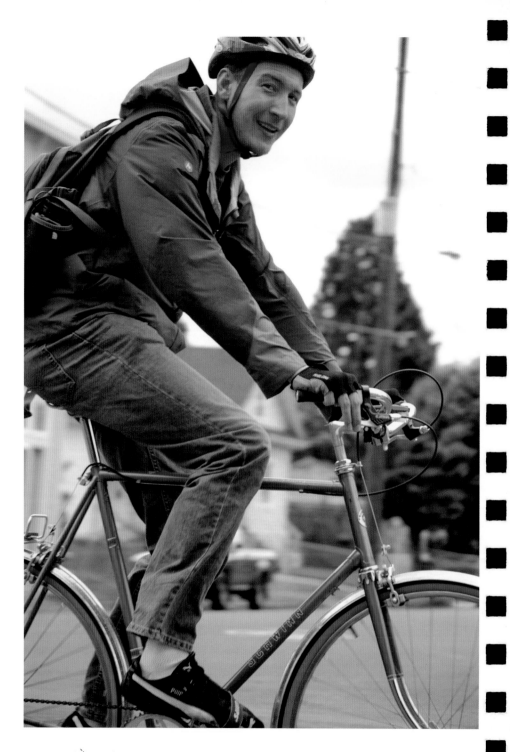

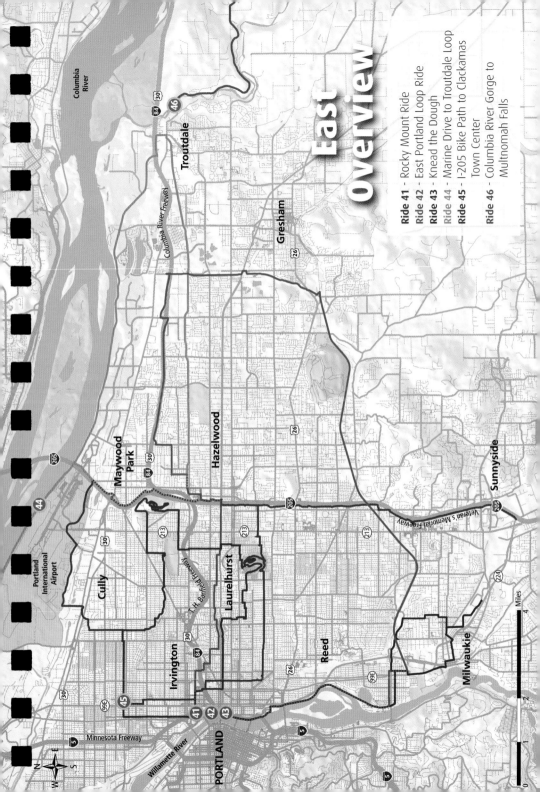

East
Overview

Ride 41 - Rocky Mount Ride
Ride 42 - East Portland Loop Ride
Ride 43 - Knead the Dough
Ride 44 - Marine Drive to Troutdale Loop
Ride 45 - I-205 Bike Path to Clackamas
         Town Center
Ride 46 - Columbia River Gorge to
         Multnomah Falls

Columbia River

Columbia River Freeway

Troutdale

Gresham

Maywood
Park

Hazelwood

Sunnyside

Portland
International
Airport

Cully

Laurelhurst

Reed

Milwaukie

Irvington

I. H. Banfield Freeway

Minnesota Freeway

PORTLAND

Willamette River

Veteran's Memorial Freeway

Miles

N
W — E
S

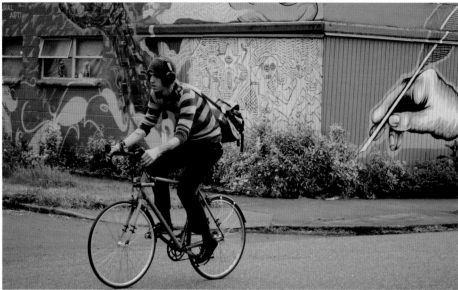

Colorful North Williams Avenue.   *Image Matt Wittmer*

At a Glance

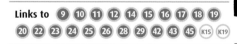

Distance 20.6 miles   **Elevation Gain** 1497′
Distance from Downtown Portland 1.2 miles

Terrain

Paved streets and bike paths.

Traffic

Urban streets, some with bike lanes and low to moderate traffic.

How to Get There

By car, take the Steel Bridge east to NE Oregon Street, left onto NE First Avenue, left onto Multnomah Street, left onto NE Wheeler Avenue; on-street parking.

By public transportation, take any TriMet MAX Red, Blue or Green train to the Rose Quarter MAX station.

Food and Drink

There is a café at the Rose Quarter MAX station and several places along the route there are neighborhood retail stores. There are restrooms and drinking fountains at Mount Tabor, but not at Rocky Butte.

Side Trip

The Grotto, a Catholic sanctuary and church, are located at the base of Rocky Butte. Services are performed in the carved out rock face and provide a cool, quiet sanctuary in the summer. During the holidays, the entire Grotto is a spectacle of lights and is a favorite of young and old alike.

Links to 9 10 11 12 14 15 16 17 18 19 20 22 23 24 25 26 28 29 42 43 45 K15 K19

Where to Bike Rating

About...

This ride takes you to two of the three extinct volcanoes within the Portland city limits. The third is Powell Butte which has unpaved pathways perfect for mountain biking. The two buttes on this ride are Rocky Butte and Mount Tabor. Rocky Butte offers a sweeping 360 degree view of Portland and surrounding areas. Mount Tabor has a popular sunset view of the city of Portland.

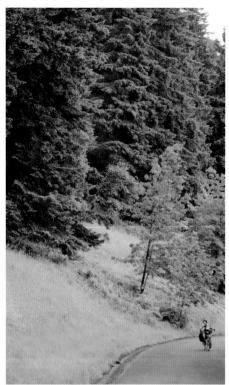

One peak down, one to go.   Image Matt Wittmer

Rocky Butte is an extinct volcanic cinder cone butte. The ride up is not as steep as it seems when you are at the bottom of the butte looking up. At the summit is the Joseph Wood Hill Park which is constructed of stone and resembles a fortress. Hill established the Hill Military Academy which is now home to the City Bible College at the base of the butte. Several of the bunkers have been renovated and are used by the college today. In the park at the summit old fashioned lights sit atop the hand carved stone wall and illuminate the park at night. Rocky Butte is a favorite of mountain climbers and there are over 150 climbing routes available. From the summit you can see the airport, the Columbia River Gorge, downtown Portland, and Vancouver.

Mount Tabor provides 196 acres of park that rises 643 feet and offers a picturesque view of downtown Portland. The climb up Mount Tabor is steeper than the climb up Rocky Butte, but you'll have lots of company as this is a popular park with cyclists. The majestic statue of Harvey Scott, a pioneer, editor, and academician, greets visitors at the summit. Five Romanesque style reservoirs were built on Mount Tabor. All but one of these reservoirs have continued to serve Portland for more than a hundred years. On the descent you will be charmed by these open water reservoirs. Mount Tabor generates its own electricity to light the historic lamp posts that follow the original roads and paths in the park and was home to the maintenance center for Portland Parks and Recreation for over a century. The site includes a large, historic plant nursery that has grown many plants, including street trees, for the city and the region. Mount Tabor was included in the National Register of Historic Places in 2004. The summit is a favorite after dinner stop for neighborhood residents who watch the sun set over the city buildings.

In addition to the long flights of stairs, gently curving parkways, and numerous walking trails, the park has basketball and tennis courts, playgrounds, picnic tables, and an amphitheater. Interested in preserving the charm of their neighborhood park, the surrounding neighborhood has successfully mounted opposition to the city's plan to bury the open reservoirs that add to the charm of the park.

East

Ride Log

0.0 From the Rose Quarter TriMet MAX station ride up NE Wheeler St.

0.2 Slight right onto N Williams Ave.

1.9 Right onto NE Going St.

3.9 Right onto the Cycle Track on NE 33rd Ave and travel along Wilshire Park.

4.0 Right onto NE 37th Ave.

4.3 Turn left onto NE Alameda St, then an immediate right to remain on NE Alameda St. (Going straight the road becomes NE Milton St.)

4.7 Right onto NE 41st Ave, and then left onto NE Beaumont St.

4.9 Right to remain on NE Alameda St.

5.3 Left to stay on NE Alameda St.

5.7 At NE Sandy Blvd make a box turn to cross diagonally and remain NE Alameda St.

6.4 Left onto NE Sacramento St.

6.5 Left onto NE 72nd Ave.

6.9 Right onto NE Fremont St.

7.9 Sharp right onto NE 92nd Ave/NE Academy Ave.

8.1 Slight right onto NE Rocky Butte Rd.

9.0 Right to circle around the peak.

9.3 Right onto NE Rocky Butte Rd through the tunnel.

10.6 Slight left onto NE 92nd Ave.

11.0 Right onto NE Tillamook St.

11.7 Left onto NE 74th Ave.

12.1 Jog right onto NE Halsey St onto NE 74th Ave.

12.8 Left onto E Burnside St.

13.1 Right onto SE 78th Ave.

13.3 Jog left at SE Stark to remain on SE 78th Ave.

13.4 Right onto SE Yamhill St.

13.6 Dogleg right at SE 76th Ave to stay on SE Yamhill St, then jog left at SE 71st to remain on Yamhill.

14.0 Left onto SE 69th Ave and enter Mt Tabor Park.

16.0 Exit the park via SE Salmon St. Cross SE 60th Ave and enter SE Salmon St through the iron posts.

16.3 Dogleg right at SE 55th Ave then back to Salmon.

16.6 Dogleg right onto SE 49th Ave and then back on SE Salmon St; dogleg left at 46th then back on Salmon.

17.0 Right onto SE 41st Ave, then right onto SE Taylor.

17.1 Left onto SE 42nd Ave, jog left at Belmont.

17.3 Left onto SE Morrison St and then right onto SE 41st Ave.

17.5 Jog right onto SE Stark St to remain on SE 41st.

17.7 Left onto SE Ankeny St and cross SE 20th Ave via a curb cut.

19.3 Right onto SE 12th Ave.

19.8 Left onto NE Lloyd Blvd, then right onto NE 11th Ave.

20.0 Left onto NE Multnomah St.

20.6 NE Wheeler Ave intersects with NE Multnomah St at the Rose Quarter. End ride.

P *P1* The Grotto

Rocky Mount Ride

Please note: the profile for Ride 41 is depicted in 200ft vertical increments due to unusually high elevation.

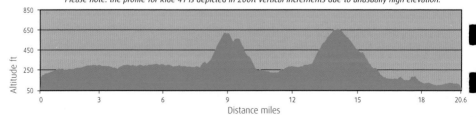

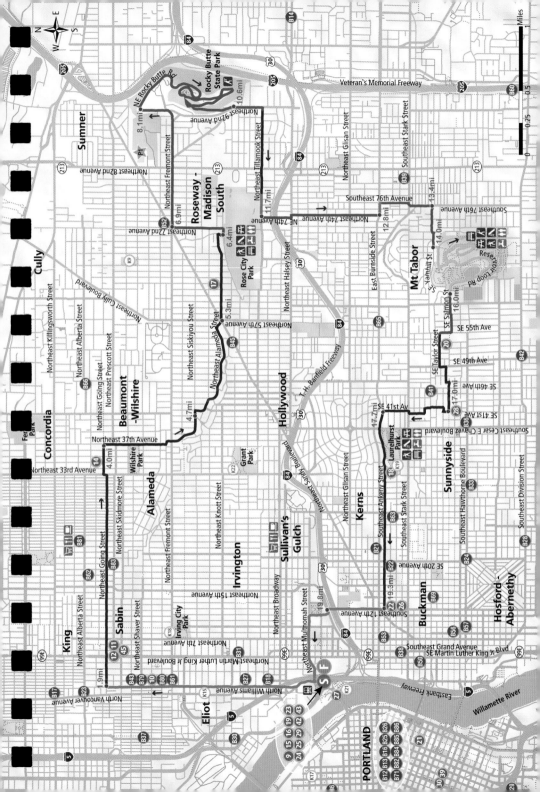

East Portland Loop Ride Ride 42

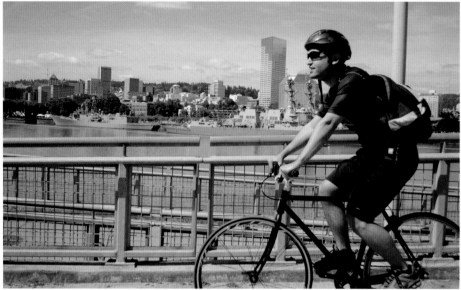

"Nothing compares to the simple pleasure of a bike ride." John F. Kennedy

Image Matt Wittmer

At a Glance
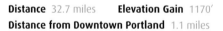

Distance 32.7 miles   **Elevation Gain** 1170′
Distance from Downtown Portland 1.1 miles

Terrain

Smooth, well-maintained streets and pathways.

Traffic

Urban and suburban, low to moderate traffic; bike paths with intersections; over half the distance is on bike and pedestrian paths.

How to Get There

By car, take Naito Parkway to the Steel Bridge east to NE Oregon Street; left onto NE First Avenue, left onto Multnomah Street, left onto NE Wheeler Avenue. On-street parking.

By public transportation, take TriMet MAX Red, Blue or Green lines to the Rose Quarter.

Food and Drink

Restrooms and drinking fountains along the Eastbank Esplanade near the Hawthorne Bridge, at the Jackson Bottom trailhead, and at Linneman station across from Club Paesano Cedarville Park. Coffee shop at the corner of the Rose Quarter MAX Transit station.

Side Trips

Oaks Amusement Park and Roller Rink, Oaks Bottom trail, downtown Sellwood for antiques shopping, Leach Botanical Gardens, Beggar Tick Wildlife Refuge, Club Paesano Cedarville Park has a playground and picnic tables.

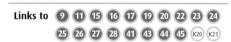

Links to 9 11 15 16 17 19 20 22 23 24 25 26 27 28 41 43 44 45 K20 K21

Where to Bike Rating

About...

The ride through east Portland brings you to the edge of the city and loops around via several bike paths that are wide and well-maintained. You'll experience the ever-popular Springwater Corridor, the new Gresham/Fairview Trail, as well as the heart-thumping I-84 bike path on your return. In between are quiet neighborhoods and lots of scenery.

Begin by riding along the Willamette River on the East Esplanade, a portion of which floats on the river. Just beyond OMSI, you'll ride through an industrial area to find the popular Springwater Corridor. You may have to take some sections slowly due to the heavy traffic.

After riding through the Sellwood neighborhood, the Goodwill Donation Center will be directly across the street in front of you as you make the left to remain on the trail. After a short distance you will travel through the Johnson Creek Watershed and Mount Hood will be framed for you by the bike path and the trees. There are several streets to cross but doing so via the pedestrian walk lights make them worry-free.

After riding past the horse farm along the back side of a residential Mount St. Helens looms in the distance ahead of you.

In Gresham, several of the street crossings have bike/pedestrian crossings and have a loud audio announcement, but no lights for cyclists indicating it is time to cross. You'll ride past the TriMet car barn, cross the tracks and ride a short distance on the street before picking up the trail again. The path will end at NE 201st Avenue. Here you will pick up the I-84 bike path halfway down the hill. Once riding alongside the highway you'll see a sign "Entering Gresham." Don't be confused! You are heading back to Portland.

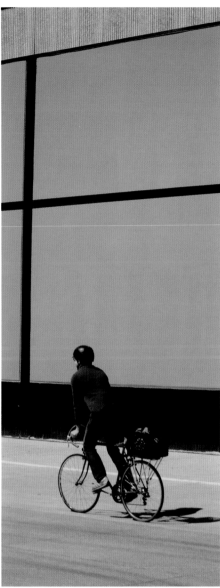

Up off the saddle near the Springwater Trail.
Image Matt Wittmer

From this point on, the ride becomes less scenic as you travel parallel to the busy highway and then onto Halsey Street. Once past these areas, you are able to slip through residential neighborhoods, making the trip much more appealing as you return to Portland.

East

Ride Log

0.0 Begin at Rose Quarter TriMet MAX station. Left onto NE Wheeler St.

0.1 Left onto NE Interstate Ave; cross at light to opposite sidewalk downhill to iron fence; right to cross bridge; left at bottom of switchbacks onto Eastbank Esplanade.

1.8 Left onto SE Caruthers St cul-de-sac.

2.0 Right onto SE Fourth Ave to Springwater Corridor gateway.

5.1 Left onto SE Spokane St.

5.9 Right on SE 19th Ave.

6.3 Left through concrete barriers onto trail toward Gresham.

16.0 Left onto Gresham/Fairview Trail at SW 10th St (unfinished street); right to continue on trail.

17.9 Left across Tri Met tracks at SE 222nd Ave on sidewalk; left onto Burnside St; ride half block to pedestrian crossing; trail is on right.

19.3 Cross NE Halsey St to continue straight onto NE 201st Ave; following signs for I-84 bike path.

19.9 Left onto access path. Left onto I-84 bike path.

21.0 Left via sidewalk; right to cross NE 181st Ave.

21.1 Left onto NE 181st Ave.

21.2 Right at second traffic light onto I-84 bike path.

24.2 Left onto NE 122nd Ave.

24.6 Right onto NE Sacramento St.

25.2 Left on NE 108th Ave.

25.6 Right onto NE Weidler St.

26.1 Left on 100th Ave at shopping center through S curve.

26.4 Right onto NE Pacific Ave; enter TriMet MAX station; follow "Bus Only" (bikes are allowed) toward fence; cross tracks; left onto bike path.

26.7 Left onto NE Glisan St over bridge; right after bridge onto bike path. Dangerous street crossing.

27.0 Right onto E Burnside St, then right onto NE 71st.

28.4 Left onto NE Davis St

29.0 Right onto NE 58th Ave, then left onto NE Everett St.

29.6 Left onto NE 47th Ave, then right onto NE Davis St.

29.9 Left onto NE 41st Ave, then right onto NE Couch St.

30.6 Right onto NE 30th Ave.

30.8 Left onto NE Glisan St.

31.2 Right onto NE 24th Ave, then left onto NE Oregon St.

31.5 Right onto NE 21st Ave.

31.7 Left onto NE Multnomah St.

32.7 Return to TriMet Rose Quarter station. End ride.

P *P1* Blue Lake Regional Park

Please note: Bike shops are not shown on this map as the scale is too large for locations to be discernable. Please see other rides in this chapter for bike shop locations.

East Portland Loop Ride

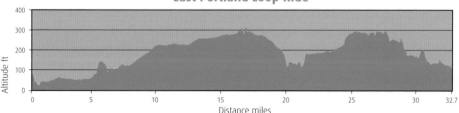

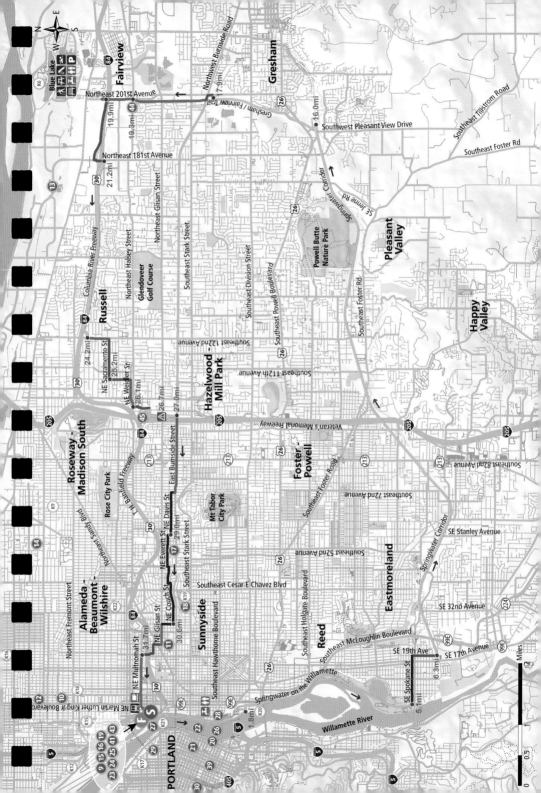

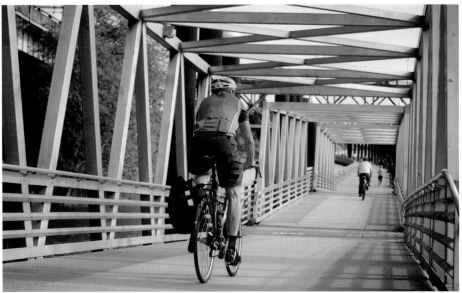

A rider approaches the floating section of the Eastbank Esplanade.

Image Matt Wittmer

At a Glance

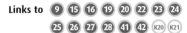

Distance 19.8 miles   **Elevation Gain** 960′

Distance from Downtown Portland 1.1 miles

Terrain

Smooth, well-maintained streets with wide bike lanes in many locations.

Traffic

Urban and suburban, low to moderate traffic; low traffic industrial park; bike and pedestrian path.

How to Get There

By car, take the Steel Bridge east to NE Oregon Street; left onto NE First Avenue, left onto Multnomah Street, left into NE Wheeler Avenue. On-street parking.

By public transportation, take TriMet MAX Red, Blue or Green line train to the Rose Quarter.

Food and Drink

Coffee shop at the corner of the Rose Quarter MAX station and numerous opportunities for refueling along the route. Be sure to save room for the goodies that await you at Bob's Red Mill and Dave's Killer Bread, the two major destinations of this ride.

Side Trips

Oaks Amusement Park, Oaks Bottom trail, downtown Sellwood for antiques shopping.

Links to 9 15 16 19 20 22 23 24 25 26 27 28 41 42 K20 K21

Where to Bike Rating

About...

Bob's Red Mill and Dave's Killer Bread, two iconic food manufacturers in Oregon, are located in Milwaukie. Beginning along the Willamette River, ride along the floating bridge of the East Esplanade, then access the ever-popular Springwater Corridor before traveling along suburban roadways to Bob's Red Mill. Dave's Killer Bread, located across the street, offers tasty samples of their robust breads. Ask to sample the Sin Dog – my favorite concoction of seeds, cinnamon, and sweetness.

The transitions between the floating section of the East Esplanade are a bit rough and very loud when you cross them. Don't be startled by the noise. The transitions are safe when you take them slowly. The path divides into two sections after you leave the floating section. Watch for pedestrians and cyclists who may be coming off the steel grid section as it rejoins the path. The East Esplanade is the best way to get to the Springwater Corridor Trail, which is very popular with all forms of non-motorized transportation including runners, cyclists, walkers, roller-bladers, and skateboarders.

Bob's Red Mill products can be found in grocery and specialty stores around Oregon and beyond. A visit to the flagship store is a wonderful treat, however, as you can wander among the amazing variety of products lining the shelves. Constructed to resemble a mill, you'll find a terrific selection of grains, legumes, and mixes. Need gluten-free products? You'll find them in bulk at the store.

Along with the wonderful selection of products you can purchase, is a cafeteria-style restaurant where they prepare food featuring Bob's Red Mill products. Select a seat inside on inclement days or outside on the patio when the weather is sunny. A pictorial history of the company is displayed on the walls.

Surrounding the building is a manicured park where visitors can wander once they have had their fill of lunch and/or snacks. Cross the street and visit Dave's Killer Bread, another Portland favorite. Here you'll find wonderful breads full of grains and seeds. My favorite part of visiting Dave's is being able to purchase items in bulk at a discount. Bring along panniers or a trailer to cart home lots of goodies.

The return ride will bring you through downtown Milwaukie along urban streets with wide bike lanes before accessing the Springwater Corridor where you'll leave motor traffic behind.

Ride Log

0.0 Rose Quarter TriMat MAX station onto green bike boxes going south toward the Steel Bridge.

0.1 Left up the hill on N Interstate Ave. Cross with the traffic light to access the opposite sidewalk.

0.2 Right just before the iron fence to access the bridge that crosses the railroad tracks. Go left down the switchbacks and left at the bottom of the ramp to head east on the Eastbank Esplanade toward Sellwood. Pass by the rear of OMSI.

2.0 Left into cul de sac at SE Caruthers. Ride through the industrial area one block.

2.1 Right onto SE Fourth Ave past the gravel elevator to the Springwater Corridor Trail Gateway.

5.4 Left onto SE Umatilla St to Sellwood.

6.1 Left onto SE 19th Ave.

6.2 Right onto SE Tacoma St.

7.0 Left onto SE Johnson Creek Blvd. SE Tacoma St ends where SE 32nd Ave and SE Johnson Creek Blvd begin.

7.5 Right at SE 42nd Ave.

8.1 Left to follow the bike path on SE Howe St one block then right on SE 43rd Ave through a residential neighborhood. The road ends at a shopping center.

8.5 Right up the hill one block, then left onto SE 42nd St around the shopping center toward downtown Milwaukie.

East

Ride Log continued ...

8.7 Right on SE Monroe St.

9.0 Left at SE 37th Ave.

9.4 Left onto SE International Way just before Highway 224. Access the left hand turn onto SE International Way through an industrial office park.

10.2 Bob's Red Mill will be on your right and Dave's Killer Bread will be on your left. Exit Bob's Red Mill parking lot left onto SE International Way.

11.1 Right at Highway 224 onto SE 37th Ave. Cross the tracks and come up the hill to the next intersection.

11.5 Left onto SE 37th Ave one block then left onto SE Oak St through downtown Milwaukie. Cross the tracks again past retail establishments. Straight through the traffic light at Highway 224.

11.9 Right at the end of the street onto SE Washington St. The road takes a sweeping turn at SE Penzance St. Turn with the road to stay on SE Washington St. High school will be on your left.

12.4 Right onto SE 21st Ave.

12.6 Left onto SE Harrison St at the stop sign. Cross over SE McLoughlin Blvd and access SE 17th Ave directly across the street. Come around the sweeping turn onto the wide bike lane. At the junction to Highway 224 beware of the right hand turn lane. Ride into the travel lane to allow the vehicles to turn right.

13.7 Right onto SE Ochoco St, cross the tracks, and down the hill one block then left at the stop sign be-

 P1 Bob's Red Mill - Dave's killer bread

tween the concrete barriers onto the cul de sac at the end of SE 19th Ave. Ride through the residential neighborhood.

14.0 Left onto SE Umatilla St.

14.8 Right onto the Springwater Corridor Trail immediately after crossing the railroad tracks at the corner of Sellwood Park.

18.0 Left onto SE Caruthers St past the Portland Opera on the right. Pick up the Eastbank Esplanade directly ahead at the end of the cul de sac.

18.2 Right to follow the Eastbank Esplanade along the Willamette River. Be sure not to miss the S curve onto the floating bridge along the river. If you continue straight, you will dead end at the stairs up to the Burnside Bridge.

19.6 Right to access the switchbacks up to the bike/pedestrian bridge that crosses the railroad tracks. Left onto the sidewalk along N Interstate Ave to the traffic light.

19.7 Left onto N Interstate Ave at the traffic light. You will be crossing with a bike traffic light that allows you to cross the street diagonally.

19.8 Right onto N Wheeler Ave, follow green bike lanes and return to the Rose Quarter Tri Met MAX station. End ride.

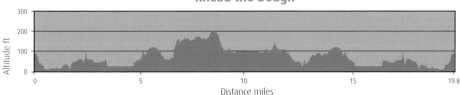

Knead the Dough

Distance miles

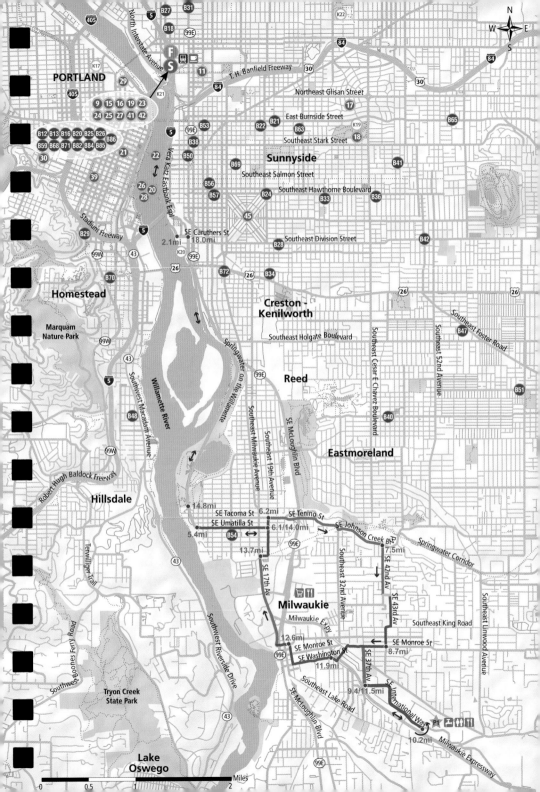

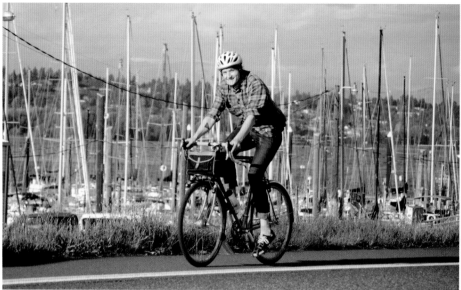

Any ride down Marine Drive delivers a best-of-book experience.

Image Matt Wittmer

At a Glance

Distance 36.4 miles **Elevation Gain** 835'
Distance from Downtown Portland 6.9 miles

Terrain

Smooth, well-maintained streets and bike paths with a short section of rough road.

Traffic

Bike paths and low-traffic streets for much of this ride with a few sections of high-traffic.

How to Get There

By car, take I- 5 N toward Seattle; take exit 307 for Oregon 99E/Marine Drive toward Delta Park; keep left at the fork, follow signs for M.L.K. Jr Blvd/Marine Drive W; turn right onto Marine Drive W. Expo Center is on the left; parking available at top of N Force Avenue or on-street.

By public transportation, take the TriMet MAX yellow line north to the Expo station, the last station.

Food and Drink

Food and restaurants can be found along the route. No public restrooms or drinking fountains.

Side Trip

Historic Troutdale, McMenamin's Edgefield, Windscape Park, Blue Lake Regional Park, and the Historic Columbia River Highway to Multnomah Falls.

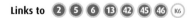

Links to 2 5 6 13 42 45 46 K6

Where to Bike Rating

About...

Ride along the dike beside the Columbia River and enjoy sweeping views of Mount Hood, the airport, marinas, and farmland. A welcome breeze off the water feels great on a warm summer day as water skiers and boaters enjoy the river. This ride takes you east to the entrance of historic Troutdale and returns you to Portland via the popular Marine Drive and I-205 bike paths. With the exception of a short section, you'll travel on multi-use paths avoiding motor traffic.

Following the Columbia River for several miles, you'll pass by Government Island, uninhabited and accessible only by boat. It is the perfect get-away on a hot summer day. Mount Hood looms ahead as you travel east passing marinas and house boats. On the day of our ride the weather had warmed enough so the snow had begun to melt on the peak.

PDX airport will be on your right. The planes taking off go directly overhead. It is quite thrilling. As you travel a bit further east you will see planes as they come in for a landing. Just before the I-205 Bridge there is a popular place to rest and watch the planes before continuing along the way.

Pass NE Blue Lake Road, the access road to Blue Lake Regional Park. Restrooms and drinking fountains are located at the park. Beyond Blue Lake the road is less traveled and the bike path crosses access roads in a couple of places. Follow the signs that direct your crossing.

Pass the Troutdale airport on your left. Along this section of road the bike lane disappears and you will come to the on and off ramps to the highway. There is a bike path that allows you to continue straight through the traffic light and under the overpass.

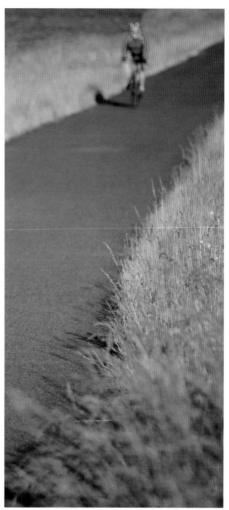

Coming into focus along the Columbia.
Image Matt Wittmer

As you enter Troutdale you will see the gateway to the Gorge on the left through historic Troutdale Center. You'll turn right to return to Portland and a short distance ahead is McMenamin's Edgefield, formerly the local "poor house" that has been converted to a popular recreation destination. The return ride along busy Halsey Street provides ample opportunity for food and beverages before returning to the I-205 bike path and Marine Drive.

East

Ride Log

 P1 Blue Lake Regional Park

0.0 From Expo MAXsStation, ride up to N Marine Dr; right onto sidewalk.

0.1 Left to cross N Marine Dr; access bike path on opposite side.

0.4 Left at sign for Marine Dr Vancouver; left onto the bike path onto N Anchor Way; ride through the cul de sac up to N Marine Dr.

0.6 Left onto N Marine Dr.

3.6 Left at the pedestrian/bike crossing onto Marine Dr bike path.

13.1 Cross N Marine Dr to continue east on roadway.

15.3 Left onto NW Frontage Rd onto highway access road via bike lane.

15.8 Right onto NE 257th Ave.

16.1 Right onto SW Halsey St. Becomes NE Halsey St.

23.7 NE Halsey St becomes NE Weidler St as a one way.

24.3 Left onto NE 102nd Ave.

24.6 Right onto NE Pacific St; cross over NE 99th Ave toward the Tri Met Gateway MAX station. Follow "Bus Only" (bikes are allowed) toward fence.

24.9 Right after tracks onto bike path.

26.3 Enter City of Maywood Park via NE Maywood

Pl - a multi-use path. Right to follow signs for Columbia Blvd; bike path ends.

27.3 Straight to cross Sandy Blvd then right to cross Columbia Blvd; ride sidewalk to access bike path on left. Follow sign for "WA points". Cross bridge over Airport Way.

28.4 At next intersection, stay straight along bike path to toward N Marine Dr.

28.6 Cross NE 112th Ave to access N Marine Dr toward Portland (left).

32.7 Cross N Marine Dr at pedestrian crossing to access bike path; under overpass bike path ends.

33.6 Right uphill parallel to NE 33rd Ave.

33.7 Left onto N Marine Dr.

34.6 Right onto NE Bridgeton Rd.

35.3 Left onto N Gantenbein Ave.

35.4 Right onto N Marine Dr.

35.7 Right onto N Anchor Way to access bike path.

36.0 Right onto bike path; cross N Marine Dr with traffic light to continue in the same direction.

36.2 Right onto opposite sidewalk

36.4 Left onto the bike path down to the Expo MAX station. End ride.

Please note: Bike shops are not shown on this map as the scale is too large for locations to be discernable. Please see other rides in this chapter for bike shop locations.

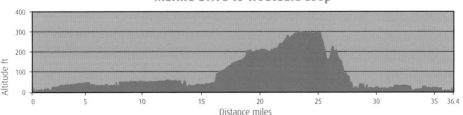
Marine Drive to Troutdale Loop

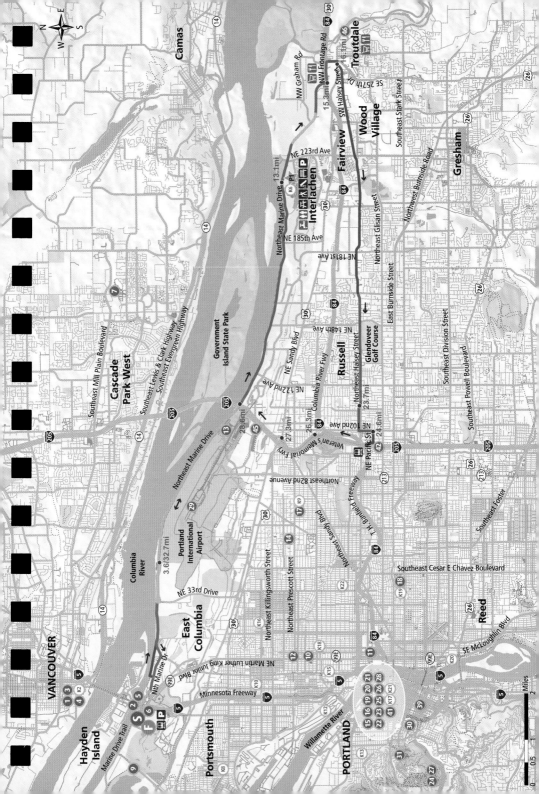

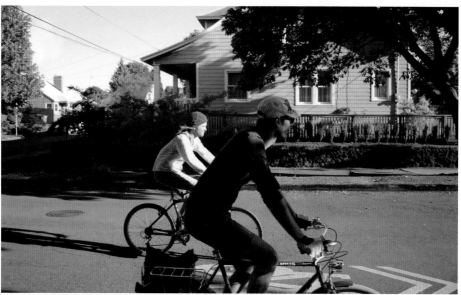

Ever-popular NE Going Street is one of Portland's designated Bicycle Boulevards.   Image Matt Wittmer

At a Glance

Distance 35.3 miles   **Elevation Gain** 1830′

Distance from Downtown Portland 4.1 miles

Terrain

Smooth, well-maintained bike path and streets.

Traffic

Bike path and low traffic streets with a couple of busy intersections.

How to Get There

By car, take the Morrison Bridge, left onto SE Grand Avenue, right onto NE Going Street. On-street parking.

By public transportation, take Bus #6 to NE Going Street and NE Martin Luther King Boulevard.

Food and Drink

There are restrooms and drinking fountains at Mount Tabor Park near the end of the ride, and many opportunities for food and drinks only short distances from this route, but none on the bike path.

Side Trip

Whitaker Ponds Nature Park is well worth a visit.

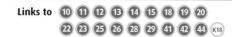

Links to (10) (11) (12) (13) (14) (15) (18) (19) (20) (22) (23) (25) (26) (28) (29) (41) (42) (44) (K18)

Where to Bike Rating

About...

Riding alongside the busy I-205 Highway without having to tangle with the traffic is a great way to travel north to south on the east side of the city. With the exception of one interruption at SE Flavel Street, another at NE Glisan Street, and several street crossings, the I-205 bike path brings the rider from northeast Portland south to Clackamas town center along this no-traffic bike path. On the return, a ride up Mount Tabor to see the city in the distance is a fitting way to end the ride.

With the incredible bicycling infrastructure around Portland, most people ride on the street along with the other vehicles. Most notably NE Going Street, where this ride begins, is one of the designated Bike Boulevards or Neighborhood Greenways. You'll find sharrows (designating a shared access roadway) painted in the street and a fair amount of bicycle traffic all hours of the day. At NE 33rd Avenue you'll ride along the short cycle track recently built by the city as a way of alleviating the difficulty of crossing this very busy street.

This ride takes you along an impressive bike path – wide and well maintained. With the exception of two small sections that take you along streets and a few intersections you'll need to cross, you can ride for miles without ever thinking about vehicular traffic. One cautionary note, however, the popularity of the Springwater Corridor makes it a major thoroughfare for non-motorized vehicles. Slow down as you approach.

The bike path can become monotonous, so on the return trip, the ride takes you off the path and through a very low-traffic neighborhood to the south side of Mount Tabor. Climb the hill to the summit and you'll have an incredible view of the city. The summit is a popular place to picnic, jog, or simply contemplate the beauty of the city from this height. On the day of our ride we met a young woman who had ridden her bike up to the summit seeking serenity, and was going to do her yoga with the city as her back-drop – the perfect setting for meditation.

After descending the extinct volcano that is Mount Tabor you'll ride through bike-friendly streets and neighborhoods, but never too far from restaurants and stores if you need food and drinks.

Ride Log

0.0 Begin at corner of NE Going St and NE MLK Blvd.

1.5 Dogleg left at NE 33rd via cycle track to remain on NE Going St.

1.8 Left onto NE 37th.

2.6 Right onto NE Holman St at Fernhill Park.

2.8 Left onto NE 42nd, bear right, cross overpass, and cross NE Columbia Blvd.

3.7 Right onto NE Cornforth St and ride along the Columbia Slough.

5.2 Left onto NE Alderwood Rd around golf course; cross NE 82nd.

7.7 At the intersection of NE Sandy and NE Columbia boulevards, cross Sandy and Columbia with pedestrian traffic lights, access bike route on opposite side riding via the sidewalk in the opposite direction of traffic.

7.8 Left to enter bike path at sign for Glisan St; do not ride over bridge; take bike path along back of bus terminal; a couple of bike paths merge with your path.

8.4 Enter the city of Maywood Park; ride through Gateway Tri-Met station.

10.5 Dogleg left at traffic light; cross train tracks via overpass; right to pick up bike path.

10.8 Right onto opposite sidewalk at NE 97th Ave and E Burnside St; cross highway overpass, left onto the bike path; ride parallel with highway; cross intersections with pedestrian traffic lights; cross Springwater Corridor.

14.8 Right at SE 92nd Ave.

East

Ride Log continued ...

15.1 Right onto Crystal Springs Blvd prior to the over-pass; left onto bike path.

15.7 Left at Foster Rd and Johnson Creek Blvd and ride under highway.

18.4 Bike path ends at SE 82nd Ave; return along same route to return to Portland.

20.1 Right at Foster Rd and Johnson Creek Blvd; ride under highway.

21.7 Right onto Crystal Springs Blvd, then left onto Flavel Rd.

21.9 Right onto bike path heading north.

25.0 Left onto Mill St and cross SE 82nd Ave.

25.7 Left onto SE 80th Ave at the Dahlia House, then right onto SE Stephens St.

26.0 Dogleg left onto SE 76th Ave; right onto SE Harrison St and enter Mount Tabor Park; ascend hill; ride through the white gate on left via bike access to reach summit; exit park via the same road.

28.9 Right onto SE Lincoln St; cross over SE 60th Ave; SE Lincoln St becomes SE Harrison St at SE 30th Ave; continue straight.

31.3 Right at the East Garden of Ladd's Addition; right onto Cypress.

31.4 Right around the Ladd's Addition Circle onto SE 16th Ave; enter the North Garden of Ladd's Addition.

31.7 Dogleg left at SE Hawthorne Blvd to remain on SE 16th Ave.

32.8 Left onto NE Irving St.

32.9 Right onto NE 12th Ave.

33.0 Left onto NE Lloyd Blvd, then right onto NE 11th Ave.

33.2 Left onto NE Multnomah St.

33.4 Right onto NE Seventh Ave.

34.7 Left onto NE Beech St, then right onto NE Grand Ave.

35.3 Left onto NE Going St one block to return to NE MLK Blvd. End ride.

Please note: Bike shops are not shown on this map as the scale is too large for locations to be discernable. Please see other rides in this chapter for bike shop locations.

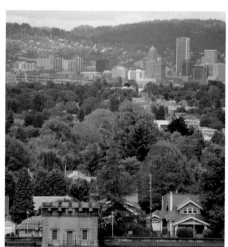

A view west off Mount Tabor toward downtown.
Image Matt Wittmer

I-205 Bike Path to Clackamas Town Center

Please note: the profile for Ride 45 is depicted in 200ft vertical increments due to unusually high elevation.

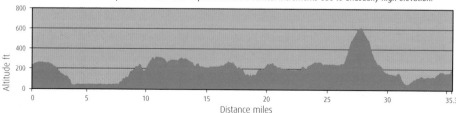

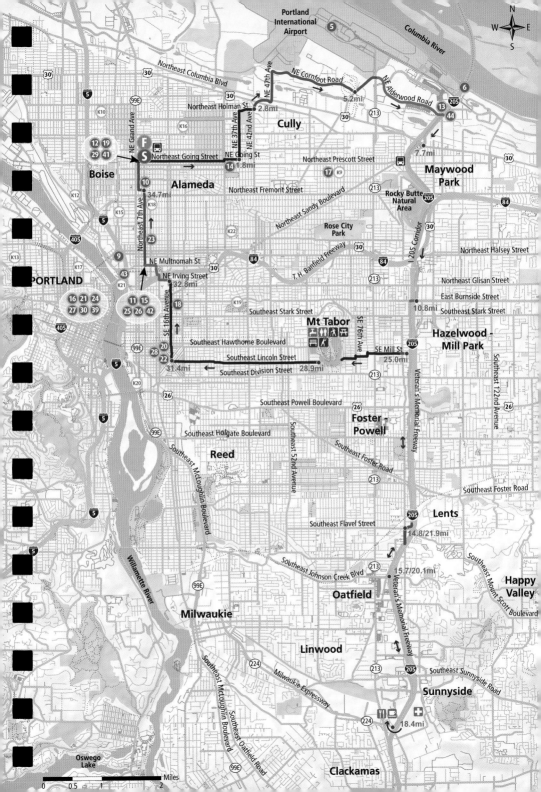

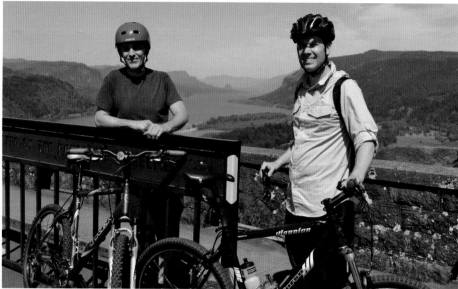

These cyclists enjoy the view of the Columbia River Gorge from Crown Point.

At a Glance

Distance 35.9 miles   **Elevation Gain** 2714'
Distance from Downtown Portland 16.9 miles

Traffic

Light traffic along the Historic Columbia River Highway.

Terrain

Varying road quality with steep drop offs and few guard rails on the return trip. This ride is recommended for experienced cyclists who are steady on their bicycles.

How to Get There

By car, I-84E/US 30-E take exit 18 toward Lewis and Clark State Park/Oxbow Regional Park; left onto Crown Point Highway, first right onto E Historic Columbia River Highway, Glenn Otto Park in on the right. Parking available.

By public transportation, take the TriMet MAX Red line east to 82nd. Board Bus #77 Broadway/Halsey to Troutdale to Glenn Otto Community Park.

Food and Drink

There are stores along the ride. At Multnomah Falls there is a gift shop and food vendors. Drinking fountains and restrooms are located at Glenn Otto Community Park, Crown Point Vista House, Bridal Veil Falls, and Multnomah Falls.

Side Trip

There are numerous opportunities to hike along the Columbia River. A ride up Larch Mountain is a good 14-mile training ride for hearty souls. Historic downtown Troutdale has several museums and unique shops. Both Oxbow and Dabney are parks worth visiting on a return trip.

Links to 44

Where to Bike Rating

About...

There are so many wonderful sights along this route that it is difficult to select just one to highlight. Though this is not the longest ride in the book, it is for experienced cyclists due to the terrain. The roads are rough and narrow, and on the return trip between Multnomah Falls and the Crown Point, there are steep drop offs along the road often with no guard rail or fence. The spectacular Oregon woods, incredible waterfalls, and sweeping vistas of the Columbia River Gorge make this ride a must.

The first landmark is Women's Forum with a sweeping vista of the Columbia River Gorge. The founding members of the Women's Forum saved this area from private development and eventually donated it to the Oregon Parks and Recreation Department. The numerous visitors to this location should be eternally grateful for their efforts.

Crown Point is next, where the octagonal Vista House is located 733 feet above the Columbia River. Continue your descent on the road that drops behind the observatory. From here the road becomes more rural and traverses through the National Forest. Next is Latourell Falls with a 224 foot plunge over the columnar basalt. Even on the hottest days of summer the short hike down the trail to Latourell Falls provides cool shade and damp spray.

Shepherd's Dell is next, but is best observed from the state park of the same name. This series of waterfalls is nestled in the woods where the rock formations curve to create several smaller waterfalls. Following is Bridal Veil Falls, which are best observed on the return ride as they descend from the creek that flows under the roadway. These falls are my favorite because they seem as delicate as the lace of a veil, thus the name. If

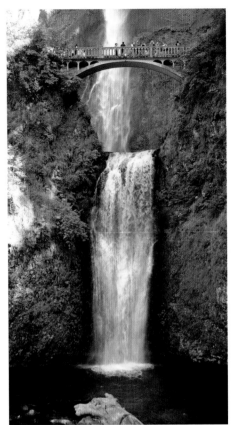

Magnificent Multnomah Falls is only one of the amazing scenic attractions along this route.

you are going to visit these falls, you will want to lock your bike at the parking lot and walk down. Be careful though, the walkway is gravel and steep in places.

The furthest point of the ride is at Multnomah Falls, the tallest waterfall in the state of Oregon. Underground springs from Larch Mountain are the year round source of this magnificent waterfall. There is a popular hike up to the bridge that crosses in front of the falls. And for ambitious visitors, the trail continues up to Larch Mountain where you can see the falls from the top of the ridge.

On the return ride, be careful of the narrow roads without shoulders. There are some sections where there are no guard rails or barriers protecting you from a precipitous drop off the side of the road.

East

Ride Log

0.0 Begin just beyond downtown historic Troutdale at Glenn Otto Community Park where there is a parking lot. Head southeast across the bridge over the Sandy River.

0.2 Right onto E Historic Columbia River Hwy/U.S. 30.

3.0 There are drinking fountains and restrooms at Dabney State Park on the right.

4.5 Turn left onto E Crown Point Hwy/E Historic Columbia River Hwy just beyond the center of Springdale; SE Hurlburt Rd is the cross street. It is busy and cyclists should take care when crossing this intersection to stay on the highway.

5.3 Slight left at SE Smith Rd to stay on E Crown Point Hwy/E Historic Columbia River Hwy.

8.5 Women's Forum is on the left side of the road; best to view the gorge from this location on the return trip.

9.0 Larch Mountain Rd veers to the right. Stay on E Crown Point Hwy/E Historic Columbia River Hwy and descend the hill to Crown Point where the Vista House is located. Enjoy the sweeping views of the Columbia River Gorge.

12.0 At the end of the winding hill is a small bridge that crosses over the stream created by the Latourell Falls. Parking is available here.

14.3 Next are the Bridal Veil Falls. The park is located on the left side of the road just before the falls. This is best viewed on the return trip.

17.2 Wahkeena Falls and lake.

18.0 Descend the last short hill to glide into Mult-

P	P1	Women's Forum
	P2	Crown Point
	P3	Vista House
	P4	Bridal Veil Falls
	P5	Wahkeena Falls
	P6	Multnomah Falls

nomah Falls. Points of interest here include the falls, the hiking trail up to the bridge across the falls, and the lodge where there are restrooms, snacks, a gift shop, and the visitor center.

21.7 Bridal Veil Falls is on the right. You will come to the falls before the parking area.

23.1 Shepherds Dell State Park has many hiking trails to explore on your return trip.

24.0 Pass by Latourell Falls just before you get ready to ascend the hill up to Crown Point and the Vista House.

27.5 Women's Forum is on your right as you descend the hill out of Crown Point. The views here of the Columbia River Gorge are magnificent.

35.9 The ride down the hill to the starting point is a wonderful descent. Be sure to be careful of debris on the side of the road and use your brakes often so that your speed does not put you in a dangerous situation. End of ride.

Note: The ride back is not as heavily traveled as the ride out to Multnomah Falls as many people who come to visit the falls take I-84 back to their destination.

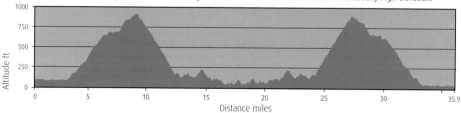

Columbia River Gorge to Multnomah Falls

Please note: the profile for Ride 46 is depicted in 250ft vertical increments due to unusually high elevation.

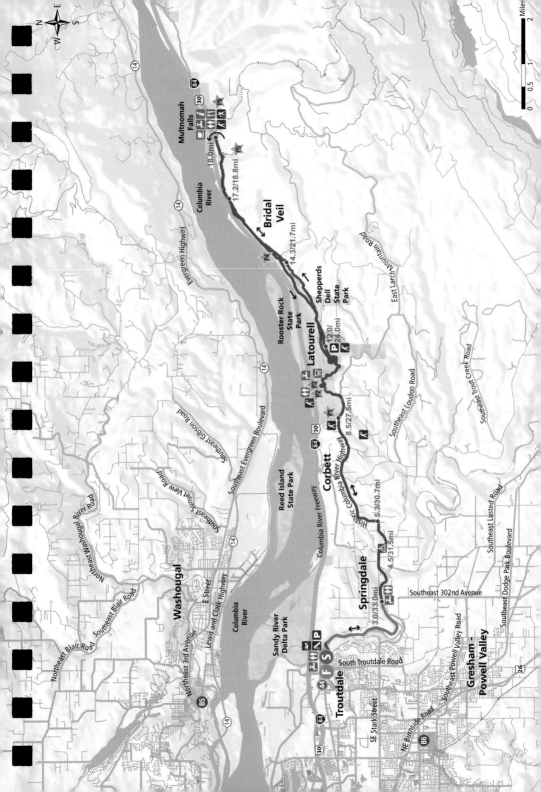

Kids' Rides

The 26 rides in this book dedicated to the youngest among us are designed to keep less confident cyclists safely tucked in areas where they will not encounter motor vehicles. Portland has an amazing array of parks and bike paths available. Many of the parks offer nature walks, play structures, picnic tables, and are closely connected to parking and shopping areas. The ones that are most conducive to the earliest cyclist and have smooth, paved pathways are included here.

Eighteen of the rides are located in Vancouver and North/Northeast Portland. Some of the bike paths are very popular family destinations. Others are in parks located within city blocks and provide places for kids to ride while adults enjoy some quiet time at a picnic table. Many of the parks have play structures and other features, such as softball fields, fountains, and disc golf courses, which are of interest to families who want to enjoy a relaxing afternoon. One of the parks even has tennis courts that are used for bike polo matches on select days of the week. While the matches are not open to young children, everyone will enjoy watching these skilled cyclists compete.

In the southeast section, where you'll find four mapped routes, is Laurelhurst Park, a popular picnic destination for many visitors and surrounding neighborhood residents alike. Consider making a trip to Grant Park, which is favored by small children who enjoy the Beverly Cleary character statues that become fountains on warm summer days. West of the city are parks with tall, old growth trees and miles of bike paths to explore. Several of the rides offered here can be extended easily for families with children who are ready for a longer ride.

The kids' rides in this book offer a variety of distances and each park has much more to offer than just bike paths, which makes them a great destination for those who want to spend time enjoying family and friends in addition to bicycling.

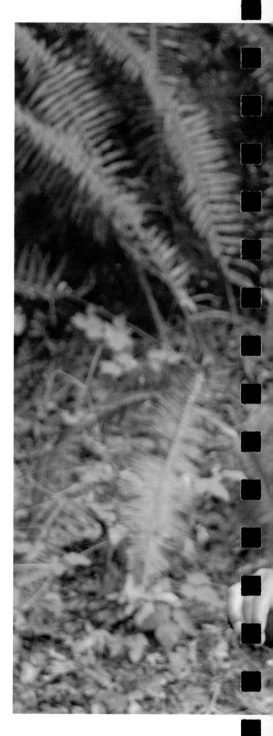

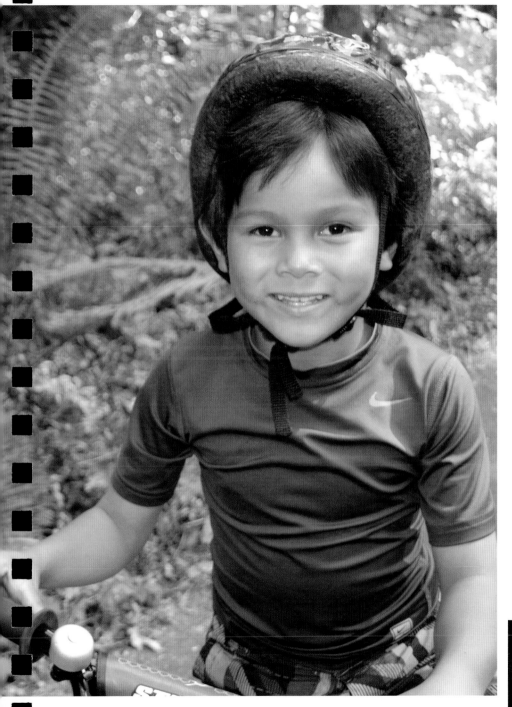

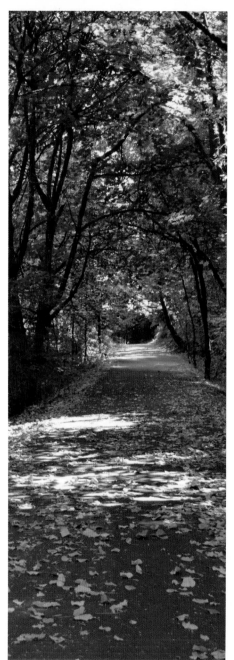

A sun-dappled path is very inviting.

Distance 3.0 miles
Distance from Downtown Portland 10.9 miles

Terrain

Paved pathways; some tree root eruptions and hills.

How to Get There

By car, take I-5 north toward Seattle; exit 2 for 39th Street; left onto E 39th Street; right onto Main Street; Second left onto NE Hazel Dell Avenue. On-street parking.

By public transportation, the trip is difficult and not recommended.

Amenities and Things to Do

There are restrooms and drinking fountains at one end of the trail.

About

Vancouver's longest continuous path, running eight miles in total length, cuts across the city via a scenic pathway through residential neighborhoods. This section of the trail can be ridden without interference from motorized vehicles and is a pleasant out and back ride through the woods. The whole family will enjoy riding alongside the creek and negotiating the hills. You'll find an abundance of tranquility on this ride through Vancouver neighborhoods.

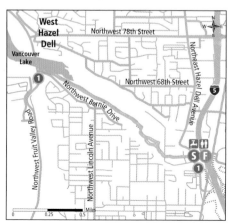

Distance 0.62 miles
Distance from Downtown Portland 8.5 miles

Terrain
Paved concrete and brick pathways.

How to Get There
By car, take I-5 north toward Seattle. After crossing the I-5 Bridge, take the second exit and follow signs to City Center. On-street parking.

By public transportation, from downtown Portland take Bus #6 to Jantzen Beach Transit Center, transfer to Bus #4 Fourth Plain Eastbound to Broadway and Seventh Street.

Amenities and Things to Do
There are wonderful shops and cafés along the streets adjacent to Esther Short Park and on weekends, there is a farmers' market on the west side of the park. Restrooms and drinking fountains are on the west side of the park.

About
Esther Short Park is a focal point of downtown Vancouver. On the corner of Columbia and Sixth streets, is the Propstra Square Glockenspiel that sits atop the 69 foot Salmon Run Bell Tower. Each hour the chimes ring and those standing close by will hear an audio story of the Chinook Indians. The park has a gazebo, wading pools, and beautiful Victorian-styled playground equipment.

This jewel of a park is a favorite of locals and offers many events throughout the year. The circular pathways are perfect for young children on their bicycles. However, because of the park's popularity and frequent events on the weekends, some of the pathways may be crowded with vendors. If you are planning on bringing your children to the park to ride, it may be wise to plan your visit for a weekday or an early morning weekend day.

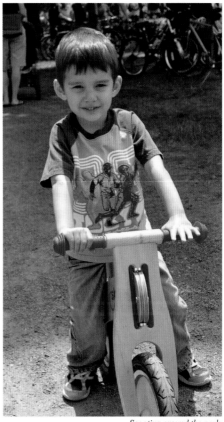

Scooting around the park.

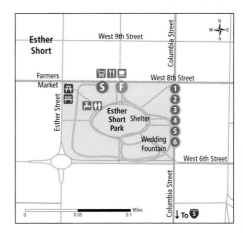

North/Northeast
Kids' Rides

Distance 2.2 miles

Distance from Downtown Portland 17.3 miles

Terrain
Smooth, paved pathways with some hills.

How to Get There
By car, take I-5 toward Seattle; take the NE 134th St E/
NE 134th Street W exit toward WSU/Vancouver; turn
right onto NE 134th Street; continue straight onto NE
Salmon Creek Avenue; WSU Campus will be on the
left.

By public transportation, the trip is very complex
and not recommended.

Amenities and Things to Do
The WSU campus has a library, walking trails, outdoor
concerts, a water fountain, a gold fish pond, and playing
fields. It is located in a residential section of Vancouver.
Restrooms and drinking fountains available but
concessions only when the university is in session.

About
A pretty ride through the center of the WSU campus
brings you to the water fountain in front of the library
and provides a wonderful view of Mount St. Helen off
in the distance. Riding down through the campus will
give you a tour of the old-growth forest and the rushing
stream that meanders through the woods.

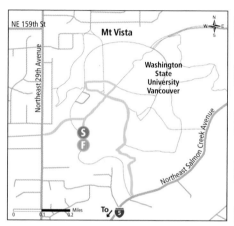

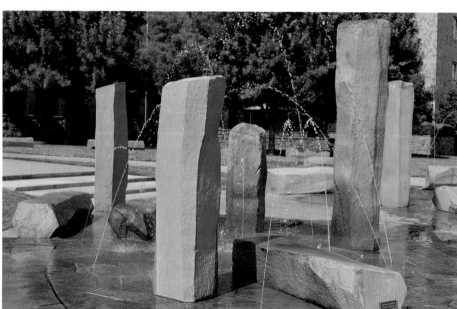

The WSU Campus is quiet and tranquil during the summer.

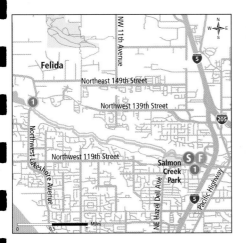

Distance 5.7 miles
Distance from Downtown Portland 12.2 miles

Terrain

Paved pathway.

How to Get There

By car, take I-5 north toward Seattle;. Take exit 3 onto NE Highway 99/Main Street toward Hazel Dell; left onto NE 63rd Street; right onto NE Hazel Dell Avenue; first left onto NE Hazel Dell Way; left to stay on NE Hazel Dell Way; continue onto NW Overlook Drive; right onto NW Dale Road. Parking available at the trailhead.

By public transportation is difficult and not recommended.

Amenities and Things to Do

Located in a residential area, the park offers restrooms and drinking fountains, picnic tables as well as play structures, a covered basketball court, an off-leash dog park, and tennis courts.

About

A great ride for both children and adults, Salmon Creek is a wonderful ride through the woods, over wooden

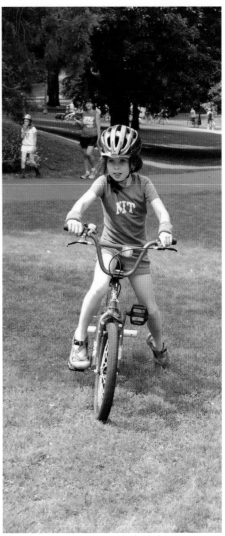

Cycling takes concentration.

bridges, and along the wetlands known as Salmon Creek. Though located in a residential and commercial area, once you are on the trail you will never know how close to civilization you are. Enjoy a leisurely ride through some of the most beautiful natural areas in Vancouver.

North/Northeast
Kids' Rides

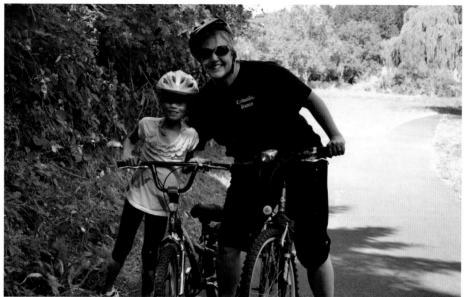

Her first ride through the woods without training wheels.

Distance 1.3 miles
Distance from Downtown Portland 11.8 miles

Terrain
Paved pathway.

How to Get There
By car, cross the Broadway Bridge; left onto SE Grand Avenue which becomes NE Martin Luther King Jr Boulevard; left onto N Marine Drive. There are two parking lots at the park.

By public transportation travel to this park is difficult and not recommended.

Amenities and Things to Do
The park offers restrooms and drinking fountains, picnic tables throughout the wooded areas as well as swimming in the river.

About
Though a distance from downtown Portland, Kelley

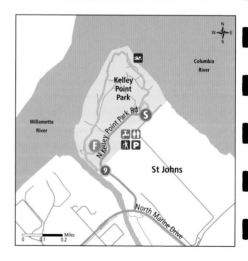

Point Park is worth the trip to sit on the river and watch the huge ships come and go. The trails wind through the woods and offer a good length and variety of sights. On the day of my visit, there was a curious raccoon peeking his nose out of the woods and the apple trees were heavy with fruit.

Ride K6 - Blue Lake Regional Park

Distance 2.2 miles

Distance from Downtown Portland 15.1 miles

Terrain

Paved, gravel, and hard-packed dirt pathways, a couple of inclines. No traffic.

How to Get There

By car, take the Morrison Bridge north, to the I-5 N/I-84 E/US-30 E ramp on the left to Seattle/The Dalles; stay on I/84 to exit 13 to Gresham, left onto NE 181st Avenue, right onto NE Sandy Boulevard, left onto NE 185th, right onto NE Marine Drive, right onto NE Blue Lake Road.

    By public transportation, take Bus #12 toward Gresham Transit Center; disembark at Stop #9775 and walk north to Fairview 1.6 miles.

Amenities and Things to Do

Several water fountains with varying sprays delight youngsters as they splash through water that gushes, dumps, and sprays. This is a popular place for boating, fishing, swimming, and picnicking.

About

This spring-fed lake is a popular place on summer days because there is plenty to keep the whole family entertained. Children under five years old are not allowed in the lake, so there are wonderful water fountains for them to play in. Rent a boat, canoe, or kayak to explore all the corners of the lake where you'll find a bevy of water lilies. The pathways allow children to explore the wetland areas while remaining close to the center of the park.

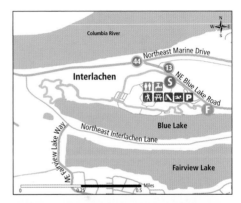

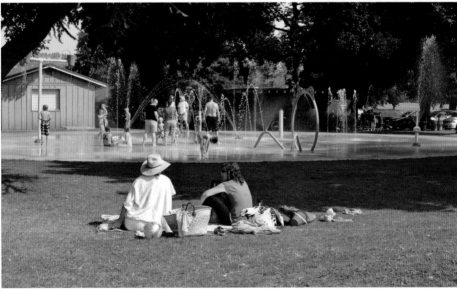

The water fountains at Blue Lake Regional Park delight children of all ages.

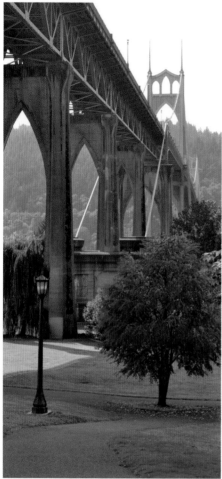

Cathedral City Park is nestled under the exquisite St Johns Bridge.

Distance 0.7 miles

Distance from Downtown Portland 8.1 miles

Terrain
Paved pathways bisected by railroad tracks.

How to Get There
By car, take U.S. Route 30 west; right over the St. Johns Bridge, continue to N Philadelphia Avenue; park will be on the left.

By public transportation, take Bus #17 to Sauvie Island via St. Johns, disembark at Stop #4440 and walk .4 miles to the park.

Amenities and Things to Do
Just steps from downtown St. Johns where you'll find restaurants and shops of all kinds, visit this park for its quiet relaxation under the majestic St. Johns Bridge. This is a great park for biking, skateboarding, picnicking, and boating.

About
The St. Johns Bridge with its cathedral-like arches traverses the Willamette River providing a unique vista for park visitors. The park is on an incline which young cyclists will find a challenging uphill climb. However, there are plenty of flat pathways at the bottom of the hill closer to the river. There is a boat launch at one end of the park, and railroad tracks bisect the park north to south. If you would rather avoid the tracks, there is plenty of space to roam on either side without having to cross over.

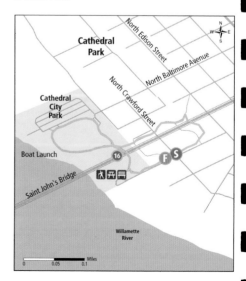

Ride K8 - Columbia Park

Distance 0.7 miles

Distance from Downtown Portland 15.7 miles

Terrain

Paved pathways. No traffic.

How to Get There

By car, take Route I/5 to exit 305B; merge onto US-30 Bypass W/N Lombard Street; right onto N Chautauqua Boulevard; second left onto N Winchell Street/ Columbia Park.

By public transportation, take Bus #4 toward St John to stop #10611.

Amenities and Things to Do

This park has lots of amenities including basketball courts, several play structures, picnic tables, water fountain, volleyball and tennis courts. Restrooms and drinking fountains are also available. Local convenience stores can provide provisions for your picnic, but there are no concessions in the park.

About

One of the oldest parks in Portland and located under

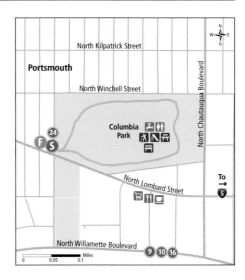

towering trees in a busy section of town, you'll find this park shady and quiet. The pathways are smooth, mostly flat and circumnavigate the perimeter of the park allowing you to stop for a picnic or to play on one of the several play structures. You'll be amazed at how quiet and serene this park is in the middle of the hubbub of the surrounding neighborhood.

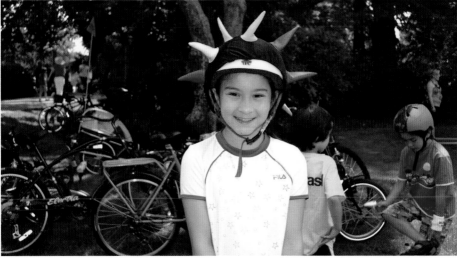

A very fancy helmet cover brings a smile to this young girl.

North/Northeast
Kids' Rides

Ride K9 - Wellington Park

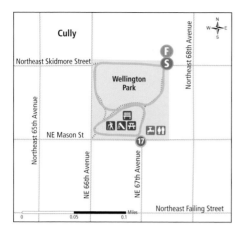

Distance 0.4 miles

Distance from Downtown Portland 7.3 miles

Terrain

Flat, paved pathways.

How to Get There

By car, take the Morrison Bridge, left on SE Grand Avenue, right on NE Fremont Street, left onto NE 66th. On-street parking.

By public transportation, take Bus #12 toward Gresham Transit Center to NE Sandy and 67th Avenue (stop #5118) and walk the short distance to Wellington Park on NE 67th Avenue.

Amenities and Things to Do

The park is located behind Harvey Scott Elementary School in a residential neighborhood. There are restrooms and drinking fountains at the park.

About

Wellington Park is a great place to teach your child to ride. A couple of the pathways are long and straight providing perfect conditions for your child to gain his or her balance and confidence. There is a water fountain and wading pool for hot summer days, and a large grassy field for a neighborhood softball game. The play area offers climbing structures and a swing set for children to play while Mom and Dad sit under the large shade trees.

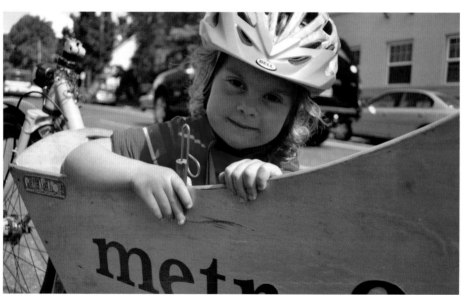

This cherub patiently awaits her cargo bike ride into the park.

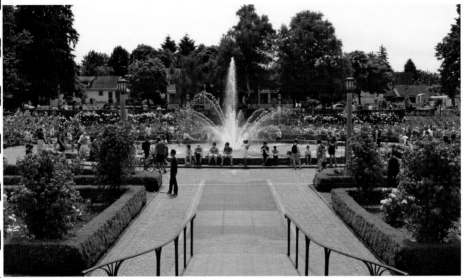

Rose gardens and fountains are a tremendous draw for summer crowds.

Distance 0.5 miles

Distance from Downtown Portland 4.4 miles

Terrain

Paved and hard-packed gravel pathways.

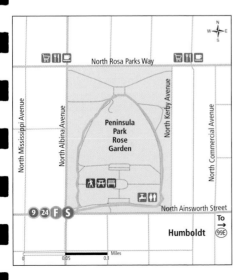

How to Get There

By car, cross the Broadway Bridge; left onto NE Grand Avenue which becomes NE Martin Luther King Jr Boulevard; left onto N Ainsworth Street to corner of N Kerby Avenue. On-street parking.

By public transportation, take Bus #44 toward St Johns; disembark at Stop #4458.

Amenities and Things to Do

Located in a residential area, the park offers restrooms and drinking fountains; includes basketball court, fountain, horseshoe pit, picnic shelter, playground, public garden, rose garden, soccer field, softball field, spray feature, stage, tennis court, and lighted tennis courts. Small convenience stores are located nearby.

About

The color and fragrance bursting forth from Peninsula Park are only a backdrop to the activities local residents enjoy at this beautiful park. Drawn by the rose garden and fountain along N Ainsworth Street, the park has much to offer families.

North/Northeast kids' rides

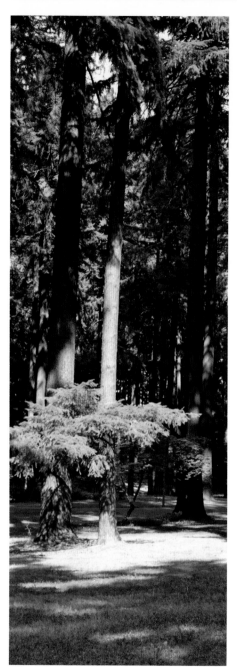

Old growth trees provide great shade on a hot day.

Distance 1.2 miles
Distance from Downtown Portland 8.5 miles

Terrain
Paved paths in play/picnic areas, and hard-packed gravel through the woods.

How to Get There
By car, take U.S. 30 west/NW St Helens Road north; slight left onto NW Bridge Street; cross St. Johns Bridge; continue onto N Philadelphia Avenue; left onto N Lombard Street; right onto Pier Park at N Bruce Avenue. On-street parking.

By public transportation, take TriMet MAX Yellow line to Lombard Transit Center, then Bus #75 toward St Johns; disembark at Stop #10697.

Amenities and Things to Do
Located in a residential area, the park offers restrooms and drinking fountains, picnic tables and shelters as well as play structures, a skate park, water fountain, playing fields, and an extensive disc golf course.

About
Pier Park is a favorite because of the variety of activities that everyone can enjoy. The topography provides challenging hills, varied terrain, and sufficient distance to entertain cyclists of all ages.

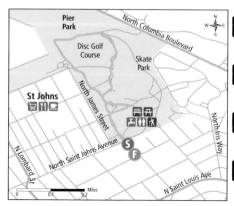

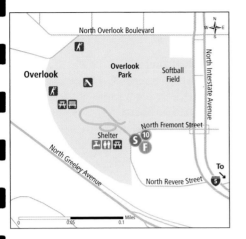

Distance 0.2 miles
Distance from Downtown Portland 2.8 miles

Terrain

Paved pathway and cedar chip pathways.

How to Get There

By car, take the Broadway Bridge east; right onto N Larrabee Avenue, right onto N Interstate Avenue, left onto N Fremont Street. On-street parking.

By public transportation, take TriMet MAX Yellow line toward the Expo Center; disembark at Stop #11510 and walk across the street to the park.

Amenities and Things to Do

Located between the Willamette River and N Interstate Avenue, Overlook Park is close to convenience stores. Inside the park you'll find a softball field, play structures, picnic tables, and a granite stone picnic shelter. Restrooms and drinking fountains are located at the picnic shelter.

About

Overlook Park provides wonderful green space along a busy section of N Interstate Avenue. There is a short paved pathway that circles both the play structure and the picnic shelter. For those with fat, treaded tires, there is a cedar chip pathway that circles the softball field. The park pathways are completely flat and are visible from almost every angle providing parents with the opportunity to give a little more freedom to young cyclists.

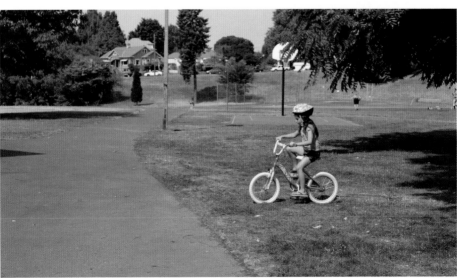

Riding on the grass is fun and bumpy.

North/Northeast Kids' Rides

Ride K13 - Wallace City Park

Distance 0.5 miles
Distance from Downtown Portland 2.3 miles

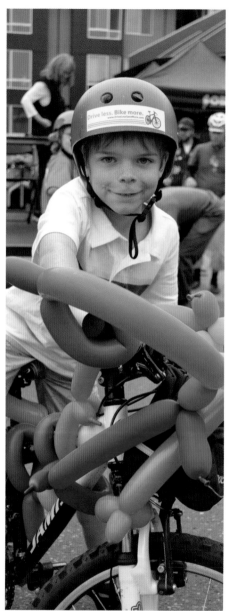

Proud of his decorated bike.

Terrain
Paved pathway; some root eruptions.

How to Get There
By car, take W Burnside Street south; right on NW 23rd Avenue; left on NW Quimby Street to NW 25th Avenue. On-street parking.

By public transportation, take Bus #15 toward Montgomery Park; disembark at NW 23rd Avenue and Raleigh Street at Stop #9031.

Amenities and Things to Do
The park offers restrooms and drinking fountains, picnic tables as well as play structures, an off-leash dog park, and tennis courts.

About
Located on the edge of downtown Portland, Wallace Park is surrounded by apartment buildings and condominiums just two blocks from NW 23rd Avenue, one of the most desirable shopping districts in the city. The pathways meander through the park and have a slight elevation to provide some challenge to young cyclists. The park is popular with young families who live in the vicinity.

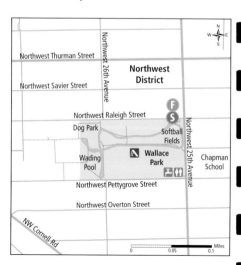

Ride K14 - McKenna Park

Distance 0.3 miles
Distance from Downtown Portland 7.8 miles

Terrain
Paved pathways. No traffic.

How to Get There
By car, take I/5 to exit 305B Lombard Street; merge onto US-30 Bypass W/N Lombard Street; left onto N Westanna Avenue; left onto N Princeton Street; park is on the left. On-street parking.

By public transportation, take Bus #35 to Stop #4491 and walk northwest 0.3 miles to the corner of N Wall Avenue and N Princeton Street.

Amenities and Things to Do
Basketball court, soccer field, picnic tables, and a softball field are surrounded by grassy parkland. There are no concessions, restrooms or drinking fountains at this park.

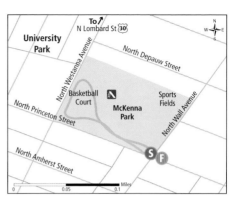

About
An inner city park, McKenna Park provides welcome green space for neighborhood children to play. Though smaller than many of the parks contained in this book, McKenna Park provides flat, paved pathways for children to learn to ride their bikes. And the basketball court is a magnet for slightly older cyclists to try out their cycling tricks.

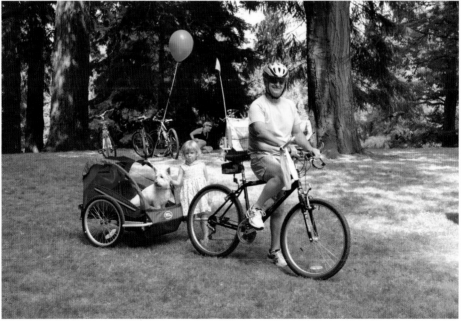

The gang is ready for the park!

North/Northeast
Kids' Rides

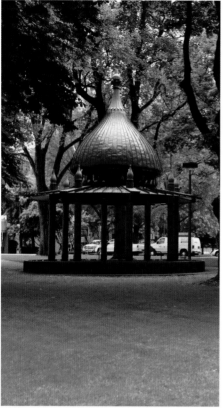

The distinctive onion-domed gazebo distinguishes Dawson Park.

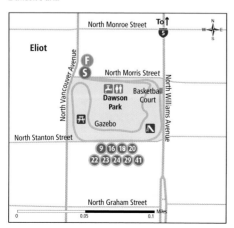

Distance 0.4 miles
Distance from Downtown Portland 1.9 miles

Terrain
Paved, flat pathways.

How to Get There
By car, take the Broadway Bridge north; left onto N Williams Street; turn left onto Dawson Park/N Morris Street. The park is on the left. On-street parking is available.

By public transportation, take either Bus #44 or #4 to NE Morris Street and walk ¼ mile south to the park.

Amenities and Things to Do
In addition to the permanent checkers tables, there is a disabled access play structure and restrooms. There are numerous opportunities for food and beverages on North Williams Avenue. Also available at the park are basketball and volleyball courts.

About
Dawson City Park is located in a diverse urban neighborhood between North Vancouver and North Williams avenues. The neighborhood has deep African-American roots. The park is a favorite gathering place on warm evenings for neighborhood residents. Expect to hear music as you approach the park as neighbors gather over picnic suppers on most weekend days. The popular play structure is at the opposite side of the park from the onion-domed gazebo. Having been rescued from the Hill Block Building, once a cornerstone of the old Albina commercial district, the dome is a distinctive element of this city park.

This park is a great place to teach children to bicycle. The flat walking paths provide the perfect terrain for the wobbly youngster learning to ride without training wheels. And when they are finished with bicycling, the play structure is a wonderful diversion.

Ride K16 - Alberta Park

Distance 0.8 miles
Distance from Downtown Portland 5.3 miles

Terrain
Paved pathway.

How to Get There
By car, cross the Broadway Bridge; left onto NE Grand Avenue which becomes NE Martin Luther King Jr Boulevard; right onto NE Killingsworth Street, left onto NE 19th Avenue. On-street parking.

By public transportation, take Bus #8 toward Middlefield Road; disembark at Stop #6792.

Amenities and Things to Do
Located in a residential area, the park offers restrooms and drinking fountains, picnic tables as well as play structures, a covered basketball court, an off-leash dog park, and tennis courts.

About
Not far from the Alberta Arts district, Alberta Park is a great place to include in your weekend plans. The play structures are very popular with children of all ages because they offer a variety of activities and the towering trees provide shade where needed. On Sunday afternoons and Wednesday evenings the tennis courts are reserved for those who wish to play bike polo – a game of skill and balance. But whatever your interest, Alberta Park is fun to visit.

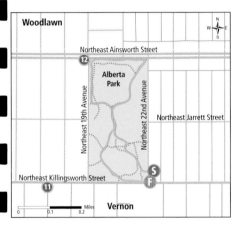

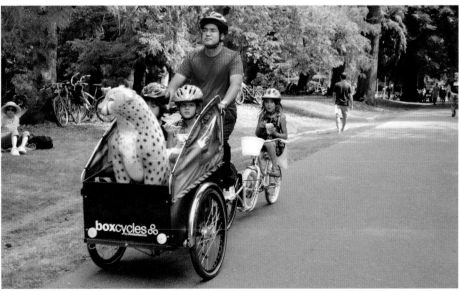

All aboard for a trip to the park!

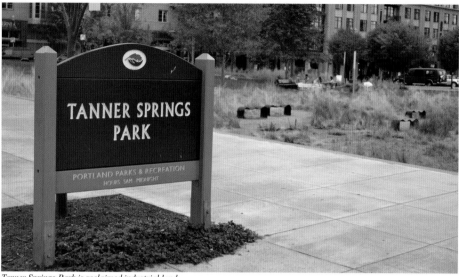

Tanner Springs Park is reclaimed industrial land.

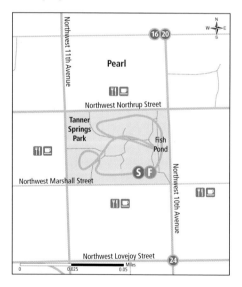

Distance 0.2 miles
Distance from Downtown Portland 0.9 miles

Terrain

Paved pathway, cobblestones, and boardwalk.

How to Get There

By car, drive northwest on SW Morrison Street toward SW Broadway, turn right onto SW 10th Avenue. On-street parking.

By public transportation, take Bus #17 toward Sauvie Island via St. Johns; disembark at the corner of NW Glisan and NW 10th Avenue at Stop #2011.

Amenities and Things to Do

Surrounded by restaurants and retail establishments, close to downtown Portland, and the waterfront.

About

Located in the desirable Pearl District this park sits in the shadow of downtown close to the waterfront. Originally an industrial complex, this reclaimed city block has been built with several unique features. Half the park is a gold fish pond surrounded by a boardwalk. Stairs and park benches provide ample areas for sitting. Opposite the pond is green space with cobblestone pathways, a bubbling brook, and gravel pathways. While there are no play structures, this space offers the young cyclist the fun of riding on varied surfaces.

Ride K18 - Irving Park

Distance 0.72 miles
Distance from Downtown Portland 3.4 miles

Terrain

Paved pathways; some tree root eruptions and hills.

How to Get There

By car, take the Morrison Bridge; left onto SE Grand Avenue which becomes NE Martin Luther King Boulevard; right onto NE Stanton Street, take the third left onto NE Ninth Avenue, .2 miles to Irving Park.

By public transportation, take the #6 along NE Martin Luther King Boulevard and walk three blocks down Fremont Street or Bus #24 runs along Fremont Street.

Amenities and Things to Do

Directly across the street from the park on Fremont Street is a vintage store, Whole Foods Supermarket, a coffee shop, pizza shop and other retail establishments are down the street to the east. The park has tennis courts, soccer field, two baseball fields, a large play structure, swings, a fountain for the children to play in, and an off-leash dog run at the top of the hill. The park abounds with picnic tables, drinking fountains, and paths that crisscross around the park for numerous variations on rides.

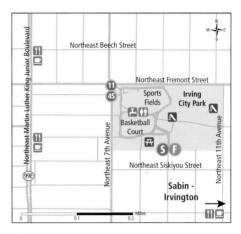

About

The land in the Irvington neighborhood was originally owned by Captain William Irving, who was famous in early Pacific Northwest maritime history and is remembered as one of the most successful and popular captains of the era. Part of the land occupied by Irving Park was the site of the Irvington Racetrack, one of four defunct racetracks now sporting Portland parks. This park is a popular place for school groups during the school year due to the baseball fields. It is also a great place for cooling off on hot summer days when the fountains are gushing water. And the tennis courts are very popular with young and old.

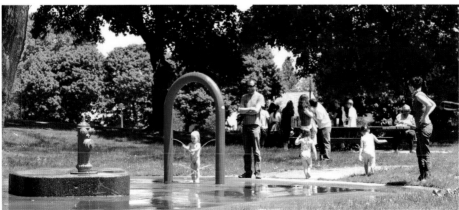

Cool fountains provide relief on hot summer days.

North/Northeast Kids' Rides

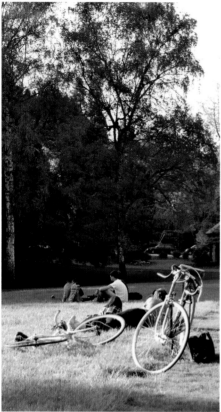

Laurelhurst Park is wildly popular with families on warm, sunny days.

Distance 0.86 miles

Distance from Downtown Portland 3.1 miles

Terrain

Paved paths, some hills, some hard-packed gravel paths.

How to Get There

By car, take the Morrison Bridge east; left onto SE Grand Avenue; right onto SE Stark Street; left onto SE 37th Avenue; right onto SE Oak Street; on-street parking.

By public transportation, take Bus #19 to NE Glison and NE 39th Avenue; walk south four blocks to the park.

Amenities and Things to Do

Laurelhurst Park is over 26 acres of beautiful woods, pond and flowering bushes in the middle of a quiet residential neighborhood. This popular park has an off-leash dog area, a large field, a pond, horseshoe pits, many picnic areas, volleyball court, basketball court, play structure, tennis courts, and a stage. The paths in the park are wide, so there is plenty of room for everyone to walk or bike

About

In 2001 Laurelhurst Park was the first city park to be named on the National Historic Register of Historical Places. This treasured park is like a second home to many during the warm summer months. The old growth trees provide a welcome shade canopy on hot afternoons. The land was originally owned by William S. Ladd who also developed Ladd's Addition and was twice elected mayor of Portland. The three acre pond in the park was at one time patrolled by a white swan whose nickname was General Pershing. He was protector of the lake and aggressively guarded his territory if anyone approached the edge of the lakeshore. After General Pershing came a black-beaked, black-toed swan named Big Boy. According to neighborhood history, a man, known only as Mr. Martinson, fed Big Boy every day for 15 years and taught him to nod his head and honk "Hello!"

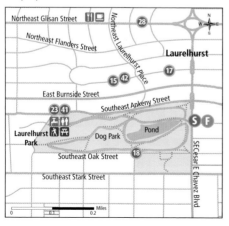

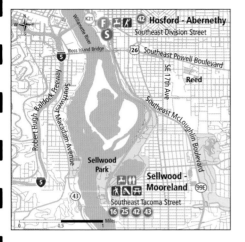

Distance 3.0 miles

Distance from Downtown Portland 1.4 miles

Terrain

Paved pathways.

How to Get There

By car, take the Hawthorne Bridge east, right onto SE Water Street. On-street parking.

By public transportation, take Bus #33 toward Oregon City to Stop #2641 on the Hawthorne Bridge.

Walk down the stairs and take a left onto the East Esplanade. OMSI (Oregon Museum of Science and Industry) is .3 miles.

Amenities and Things to Do

Restrooms and drinking fountains can be found just before the Hawthorne Bridge and at Sellwood Park. Oak Park Amusement Park and Oak Park Roller Skating Rink are located just before Sellwood Park. There are also several areas where unpaved paths bring you closer to the water or into the wooded nature trails.

About

Beginning on the East Esplanade at OMSI, this ride takes you along the Springwater Corridor to Sellwood Park. This is one of the most popular bike and pedestrian pathways in the city. Though it is free of motor vehicles, it has a plethora of other traffic including skateboarders, pedestrians, cyclists, and roller skaters. On a sunny weekend day, there can actually be traffic jams. Because of the heavy traffic, I would recommend this ride for children who are slightly older and confident cyclists. If you must bring young children, plan for an early visit to avoid the crowds.

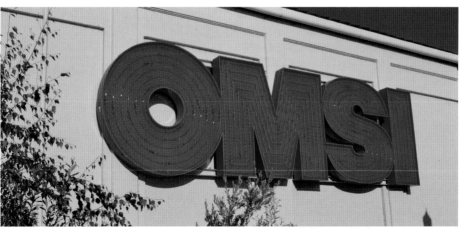

OMSI is one of the biggest museums around.

Distance 2.95 miles
Distance from Downtown Portland 1.4 miles

Terrain
Paved pathways and floating bridges.

How to Get There
By car, taking the Hawthorne Bridge east, then right onto SE Water Street. On-street parking.

By public transportation, take any MAX train to the Rose Quarter. Walk southwest to the Steel Bridge, or take the Red or Blue line to Old Town/Chinatown MAX station and walk to the river front.

Amenities and Things to Do
The East Esplanade is located on the Willamette River between the Steel Bridge and OMSI (Oregon Museum of Science and Industry). There are numerous places to stop and sit on park benches. Restrooms and drinking fountains can be found just after the Hawthorne Bridge. Visit OMSI, the Oregon Maritime Museum, feed the ducks, or rent a pedi-cab.

About
This popular section of the Willamette River offers breathtaking views of the city. One section of the bridge floats on the Willamette River. There are two steel bridges that connect the floating portion to the land-based portions. Riding over the bridges can be loud and slippery when wet. Depending upon the height of the river, the bridges create varying angles of incline, and can be loud when riding over them.

Stop at the statue of Vera Katz, former mayor and champion of the East Esplanade pathway. You'll find her statue sitting on a cement wall just before the Hawthorne Bridge. This trip will not be complete without a visit to OMSI, one of the best museums anywhere. *Please note: since Kids Ride 21 is located adjacent to Downtown Portland, there are too many links to adult rides to show them on the map above.*

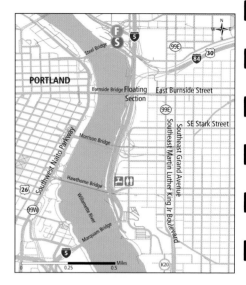

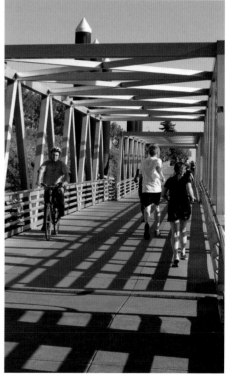

The floating section of the East Esplanade.

Distance 0.84 miles
Distance from Downtown Portland 3.7 miles

Terrain

Smooth pathways and slight hills.

How to Get There

By car, take I-84 E/US-30 East to exit #1 for 33rd Avenue; turn left onto NE 33rd; Grant Park is .5 miles. The best entry point is NE 36th Avenue and NE Brazee Street where there is on-street parking.

By public transportation, take Bus #73 toward Sunderland.

Amenities and Things to Do

The park is adjacent to Grant High School. Lit tennis courts occupy the middle of the park, next to which you'll find drinking fountains and restrooms. As you enter from NE 36th and NE Brazee Street, the off-leash dog run area is on the left. Grant Park also has a running track, play structure, and several basketball courts. This is a quiet residential neighborhood, but travel three or four blocks in any direction and you will find coffee shops, restaurants and other retail stores.

About

Grant Park was named in honor of President Ulysses S. Grant, but the real attraction here is the Beverly Cleary Sculpture Garden for Children. Sculptor Lee Hunt created the likenesses of the three Cleary characters: Ramona Quimby, Henry Huggins, and Ribsy (Henry's dog) in clay and then had them bronzed. Grant Park is only a few blocks away from Klickitat Street, which was the fictional home of the characters. There is a fountain under the feet of each figure and when the weather is hot, the city turns on the sprinklers for the children to enjoy. The sculpture garden is just south of the playground along NE 33rd Avenue.

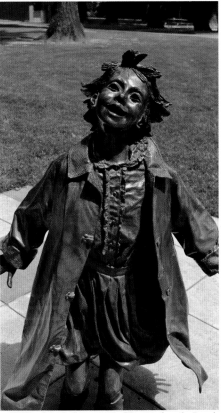

Children love the brass statue of Ramona from the Beverly Cleary novels that becomes a fountain in the summer.

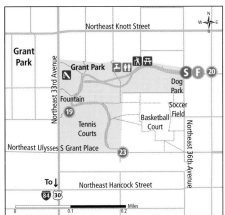

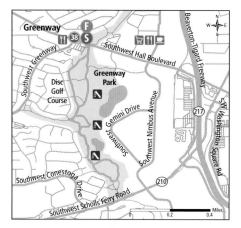

Distance 2.2 miles
Distance from Downtown Portland 10.9 miles

Terrain

Paved pathways and wooden bridges.

How to Get There

By car, take US 26W to exit 26A and merge into Highway 217W. Take exit 4A for Hall Boulevard; right onto SW Hall Boulevard; left onto SW Greenway Boulevard. On-street parking.

By public transportation, take TriMet MAX Red or Blue line to Beaverton Transit Center; transfer to Bus #78 toward Lake Oswego to Stop #2283.

Amenities and Things to Do

The park has no restrooms or drinking fountains. There are numerous places to purchase food and drinks outside the park, however. Just prior to entering the park, there is a shopping center.

About

Tucked among busy Beaverton streets and is a portion of Fanno Creek Park. Greenway Park has miles of paved pathways designed for both bikes and pedestrians to enjoy. There are several playgrounds, basketball courts, and swing sets located along the paths. The park also offers a challenging disc golf course that is quite popular and on the day of my visit there were some serious competitors on the course. There are open expanses of grassy fields begging for family picnics and impromptu softball games.

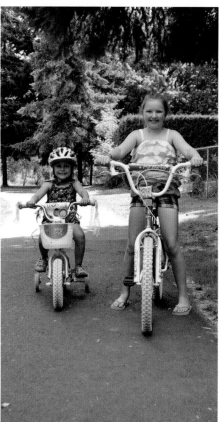

Two girls enjoying the ride on a sunny day.

Ride K24 - Tualatin Hills Nature Park

Distance 2.5 miles
Distance from Downtown Portland 10.2 miles

Terrain

Paved pathways and wooden bridges.

How to Get There

By car, take the Tualatin Valley Highway to SW Milliken Way at SW 160th Avenue. The park will be on the right. On-site parking.

By public transportation, take TriMet MAX Red or Blue line toward Hillsboro to the Merlo Rd/158th Avenue station. The park can be accessed directly across the street from the station.

Amenities and Things to Do

From the parking lot, the visitor center has restrooms, water fountains, and trail maps in both Spanish and English. Unpaved, narrow walking trails off the paved pathways. There are no concessions at the park.

About

The Tualatin Hills Nature Park is hidden behind a corporate industrial park and is a welcome sanctuary nestled in this bustling section of Beaverton. Information panels along the paths identify the plants, trees, flowers, and birds in the forest. The park has a wonderfully thick tree canopy and the pathways twist and turn. Very small children may need a helping hand to ascend the hills, but delight in the downhills. The bridges are fun to ride because the turns are tight and riding over the wood is loud! On the day of my ride there were several small boys who especially enjoyed this section of the park challenging each other to be the loudest riders on the wooden bridges.

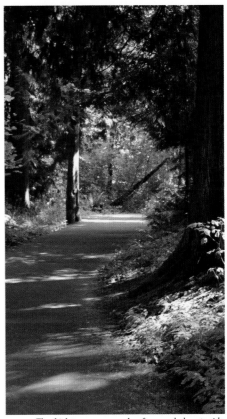

The thick tree canopy makes for a cool place to ride.

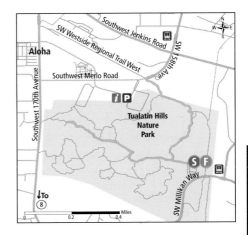

West
Kids' Rides

Distance 0.55 miles
Distance from downtown Portland 16.9 miles

Terrain
Smooth bike and pedestrian paths.

How to Get There
By car, take exit 2A off OR-217S toward Beaverton for Route OR-8 west toward Beaverton; continue 9.2 miles to destination.

By public transportation, take TriMet MAX Blue or Red line to the Beaverton Transit Center; board Bus 57 to Forest Grove; get off at 10th and Maple streets and walk northwest to Shute Park.

Amenities and Things to Do
Thirteen-acre Shute Park is the oldest park in Hillsboro. It includes not only the recreation and sports areas, but encompasses an aquatic center, the Hillsboro Library, and a community senior center. The park is located close to Hillsboro center for convenient access to restaurants and stores. A popular play structure, picnic areas, performance platform, and pickle ball court provide fun for the whole family.

About
Fiberglass statues of the A&W Burger Family sit at the entrance. These remnants from the 1960s drive-in era were placed here in 1983 having spent time promoting the A&W restaurants and, more recently, a pizza parlor.

With its tall old trees, Shute Park is a fitting place for the second statue, Chief Kno-Tah. The statue was carved by Hungarian-born Peter Toth in 1987 out of a 25 foot Douglas Fir tree weighing 33,000 pounds and believed to be approximately 400 years old.

Flat, winding pathways throughout the park give young cyclists the opportunity to explore and still be under the watchful eye of parents. On the day of my ride a young girl was thoroughly enjoying riding around winding bike paths with her Dad in hot pursuit.

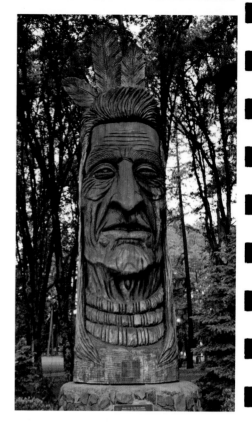

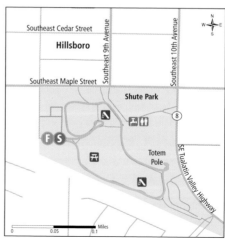

Distance 1.1 miles

Distance from Downtown Portland 15.7 miles

Terrain

Paved pathways and wooden bridges. No traffic.

How to Get There

By car, take OR 8W (also known as Tualatin Valley Highway); left onto SE Brookwood Avenue, cross the railroad tracks, immediate right onto SE Witch Hazel Road; right onto SE River Road, left onto SE Rood Bridge Road; left at Hillsboro High School to continue on SE Rood Bridge Road. On-site parking.

By public transportation, take TriMet MAX Red or Blue line to Beaverton Transit Center. Take Bus #57 toward Forest Grove; disembark at Stop #5612 and walk south on SE Rood Bridge Road 1.1 miles.

Amenities and Things to Do

Miles of paved pathways, unpaved walking trails, a pond, stream, picnic shelters, tennis courts, a boat ramp, and a large play structure. It is also home to the Lloyd Baron Rhododendron Garden. There are restrooms and drinking fountains at the park.

About

Pathways are paved and meander through the woods, with short, steep hills which may be challenging for some. The park is a very popular place for family picnics and the large play structures attract children of all ages. The interior is a wonderful place to find shade while riding on a hot summer day. Numerous unpaved walking trails run perpendicular to the paved pathways. On the day of my visit there were several families picnicking on the grassy fields. If you are looking for solitude, the Lloyd Baron Rhododendron Garden offers a quiet place to sit.

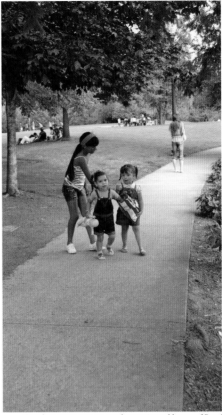

Families enjoy picnics on the manicured lawns of Rood Bridge Park.

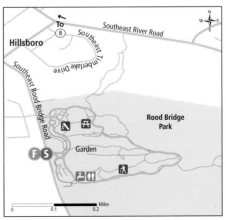

West
Kids' Rides

Notes

Notes

Notes

Notes

B1   The Bike Gallery - Beaverton
     12345 SW Canyon Road, BEAVERTON
     Tel: 503-641-2580
     www.bikegallery.com

B2   Performance Bicycle - Beaverton
     3850 SW Hall Blvd, Hall Street Shopping Center
     BEAVERTON
     Tel: 503-644-3246
     www.performancebike.com

B3   Beaverton Bike N Hike
     10120 S.W. Beaverton-Hillsdale Highway, BEAVERTON
     Tel: 503-646-6363
     www.bikenhike.com

B4   Sunset Cycles
     15320 NW Central Drive, Suite D-1, BEAVERTON
     Tel: 503-579-9264
     www.sunsetcyclesnw.com

B5   Camas Bike and Sport
     240 NE 3rd Avenue, CAMAS
     Tel: 360-210-5160
     www.camasbikes.com

B6   Gresham Bicycle Center
     567 Northeast 8th Street, GRESHAM
     Tel: 503-661-2453
     www.greshambike.com

B7   Clackamas Cycle World
     11493 SE 82nd Avenue, HAPPY VALLEY
     Tel: 503-653-5390
     www.clackamascyclewtorld.com

B8   Hillsboro Bike N Hike
     156 S.E. 4th Avenue, HILLSBORO
     Tel: 503-681-0594
     www.bikenhike.com

B9   The Bike Gallery - Lake Oswego
     200 B Avenue, LAKE OSWEGO
     Tel: 503-636-1600
     www.bikegallery.com

B10 Lakeside Bicycles
     428 N State Street, LAKE OSWEGO
     Tel: 503-699-8665

B11 Milwaukie Bike N Hike
     15080 S.E. McLoughlin Blvd, MILWAUKIE
     Tel: 503-653-2742
     www.bikenhike.com

B12 Waterfront Bicycles
     10 SW Ash Street, PORTLAND
     Tel: 503-227-1719
     www.waterfrontbikes.com

B13 The Bike Gallery - Downtown
     1001 SW 10th Avenue, PORTLAND
     Tel: 503-222-3821
     www.bikegallery.com

B14 The Outer Rim
     10625 NE Halsey Street, PORTLAND
     Tel: 503-278-3235
     www.outerrimbicycles.com

B15 The Bike Gallery - Division
     10950 SE Division Street, PORTLAND
     Tel: 503-254-2663
     www.bikegallery.com

B16 West End Bikes PDX
     1111 SW Stark Street, PORTLAND
     Tel: 503-208-2933
     www.westendbikespdx.com

B17 Cascade Cycling
     122 N Killingsworth Street, PORTLAND
     Tel: 503-281-0255
     www.cascadecycling.com

B18 Portland Design Works
     15 NE Hancock Street, PORTLAND
     Tel: 503-234-7257
     www.ridepdw.com

B19 Randall''s Family Bicycle Center
     16165 SW Pacific Highway, PORTLAND
     Tel: 503-620-1107

B20 Performance Bicycle Shop Portland
     1736 SW Alder Street, PORTLAND
     Tel: 503-224-0297
     www.performancebike.com

B21 Universal Cycles
     2202 East Burnside Street, PORTLAND
     Tel: 503-943-6152
     www.universalcycles.com

B22 Citybikes Workers Cooperative - Repair Shop
     1914 SE Ankeny Street, PORTLAND
     Tel: 503-239-0553
     www.citybikes.coop

B23 The eBike Store
     201 N Alberta Street, PORTLAND
     Tel: 503-360.-432
     www.ebikestore.com

B24 Coventry Cycle Works
2025 SE Hawthorne Boulevard, PORTLAND
Tel: 503-230-7723
www.coventrycycle.com

B25 Veloshop
142 NW 17th Avenue, PORTLAND
Tel: 503-335-8356
www.veloshop.org

B26 Bike Central
220 SW 1st Avenue, PORTLAND
Tel: 503-227-4439
www.bike-central.com

B27 Metropolis Cycle Repair
2249 N Williams Avenue, PORTLAND
Tel: 503-287-7116
www.metropoliscycles.com

B28 A Better Cycle
2324 SE Division Street, PORTLAND
Tel: 503-265-8595
www.abettercycle.com

B29 Bumblebee Bicycle
2331 SW 6th Avenue, PORTLAND
Tel: 360-936-1738
www.bumblebeebike.com

B30 Green Garage Bicycle Repair
2410 N Mississippi Avenue, PORTLAND
Tel: 971-227-4799

B31 Cycle Path
2436 NE Martin Luther King Boulevard, PORTLAND
Tel: 503-281-0485
www.cyclepathnw.com

B32 Fat Tire Farm Mountain Bike Company
2714 NW Thurman Street, PORTLAND
Tel: 503-222-3276
www.fattirefarm.com

B33 Veloce Bicycles *(Rentals available)*
3202 SE Hawthorne Boulevard, PORTLAND
Tel: 503-234-8400
www.velocebicycles.com

B34 Seven Corners Cycles
3218 SE 21st Avenue, PORTLAND
Tel: 503-230-0317
www.7-corners.com

B35 Southwest Bicycle
3605 SW Multnomah Boulevard, PORTLAND
Tel: 503-246-0333

B36 Joe Bike (USA)
3953 SE Hawthorne Boulevard, PORTLAND
Tel: 503-232-1107
www.joe-bike.com

B37 North Portland Bike Works
3978 N Mississippi Avenue, PORTLAND
Tel: 503-287-1098
www.northportlandbikeworks.org

B38 Bike N Hike Portland
400 SE Grand Avenue, PORTLAND
Tel: 503-736 1074
www.bikenhike.com

B39 Oregon Bike Shop
418 SE 81st Avenue, PORTLAND
Tel: 503-575-1804
www.oregonbikeshop.com

B40 The Bike Gallery - Woodstock
4235 SE Woodstock Boulevard, PORTLAND
Tel: 503-774-3531
www.bikegallery.com

B41 Bicycle Repair Collective
4438 SE Belmont Street, PORTLAND
Tel: 503-233-0564
www.bicyclerepaircol.net

B42 Lucky 13 Bikes
5020 SE Division Street, PORTLAND
Tel: 503-234-1313
www.lucky13bikes.com

B43 United Bicycle Institute
3961 N Willians Avenue, PORTLAND
Tel: 541-488-1121
www.bikeschool.com

B44 Hollywood Cycling
5258 NE Sandy Boulevard, PORTLAND
Tel: 503-281-1671
www.hollywoodcycling.com

B45 The Bike Gallery - Hollywood (Headquarters)
5329 NE Sandy Boulevard, PORTLAND
Tel: 503-281-9800
www.bikegallery.com

B46 Bike Tires Direct
5741 NE 87th Avenue, PORTLAND
Tel: 800-682-0570
www.biketiresdirect.com

Bike Shops & Rentals

B47 Meticon Bikes
     5925 SE Foster Road, PORTLAND
     Tel: 503-771-1737
     www.meticonbikes.com

B48 En Selle The Road Bike Shop
     6200 SW Virginia Street, Suite 202, PORTLAND
     Tel: 503-244-6754

B49 Revolver Bikes
     6509 N Interstate Avenue, PORTLAND
     Tel: 503-285-1084
     www.revolverbikes.com

B50 River City Bicycles
     706 SE Martin Luther King Boulevard, PORTLAND
     Tel: 503-233-5973
     www.rivercitybicycles.com

B51 BackPedal Cycle Works
     7126 SE Harold Street, PORTLAND
     Tel: 503-891-9842
     www.bpcycleworks.com

B52 The Missing Link
     7215 NE Sandy Boulevard, PORTLAND
     Tel: 503-740-3539

B53 Citybikes Workers Cooperative - Annex
     734 SE Ankeny, PORTLAND
     Tel: 503-239-6951
     www.citybikes.coop

B54 Sellwood Cycle Repair *(Rentals available)*
     8301 SE 13th Avenue, PORTLAND
     Tel: 503-233-9392
     www.sellwoodcycle.com

B55 Weirs Cyclery
     8247 N Lombard Avenue, PORTLAND
     Tel: 503-283-3883
     www.weirscyclery.com

B56 A Convenient Cycle
     833 SE Main Street, PORTLAND
     Tel: 503 267 8284
     www.aconvenientcycle.com

B57 Clever Cycles
     908 SE Hawthorne Boulevard, PORTLAND
     Tel: 503-334-1560
     www.clevercycles.com

B58 UpCycles
     911 NE Dekum Street, PORTLAND
     Tel: 503-388-0305

B59 21st Avenue Bicycles
     916 NW 21st Avenue, PORTLAND
     Tel: 503-222-2851
     www.21stbikes.com

B60 Performance Bicycle - Portland
     9988 SE Washington Street, Mall 205, PORTLAND
     Tel: 503-408-8150
     www.performancebike.com

B61 Abraham Fixes Bikes
     3508 N Williams Avenue, PORTLAND
     Tel: 503-953-5260
     www.abrahamfixesbikes.com

B62 Community Cycling Center
     1700 NE Alberta Street, PORTLAND
     Tel: 503-287-8786
     www.communitycyclingcenter.org

B63 Crank
     2725 SE Ash Street, PORTLAND
     Tel: 503-610-8356
     ww.crankpdx.com

B64 Cycology Mobile Bike Repair
     6718 Southeast 136th Avenue, PORTLAND
     Tel: 503-984-6658

B65 Cyclopedia
     5711 E Burnside, Suite B, PORTLAND
     Tel: 503-308-1245
     www.portlandcyclopedia.com

B66 Metrofeit Cycles
     4613 Northeast Alberta Street, PORTLAND
     PORTLAND
     Tel: 503-318-9810
     www.metrofeits.com

B67 Performance Bicycle - Downtown
     1736 SW Alder Street, PORTLAND
     Tel: 503-224-0297
     www.performancebike.com

B68 REI
     1405 NW Johnson Street, PORTLAND
     Tel: 503-221-1938
     www.rei.com

B69 Splendid Cycles
     1407 SE Belmont Street, PORTLAND
     Tel: 503-954-2620
     www.splendidcycles.com

B70 The Go By Bike Shop
SW Gibbs & Moody, PORTLAND
Tel: 971-271-9270
www.gobybikepdx.com

B71 Recyclery
730 SW 11th Avenue, PORTLAND
Tel: 503-222-1169
www.therecycelry.com

B72 WTF Bikes
3117 SE Milwaukie Avenue, PORTLAND
Tel: 503-232-4WTF (4983)
www.wtfbikes.net

B73 Tigard Cycle & Ski Service
12551 SW Main Street, TIGARD
Tel: 503-639-1000

B74 REI
7410 SW Bridgeport Rd, TIGARD
Tel: 503-624-8600
www.rei.com

B75 Performance Bicycle - Tualatin
7071 SW Nyberg Street, Nyberg Woods Shopping
Center, TUALATIN
Tel: 503-639-2522
www.performancebike.com

B76 Bad Monkey Bikes Boards and Skates
1717 Broadway, VANCOUVER
Tel: 360-718-7837
www.badmonkeybikes.com

B77 Bad Boyz Bicycle and Specialities
19002 Southeast 15th Street, VANCOUVER
Tel: 360-892-5281
www.badboyzbicycles.com

B78 Vancouver Cyclery
10108 NE Hwy 99 , VANCOUVER
Tel: 360-574-5717
www.vancouvercycleryinc.com

Bike-related Businesses

B79 Hopworks BikeBar
3947 N Williams Avenue, PORTLAND
Tel: 503-287-6258
www.hopworksbeer.com
Restaurant/bar

B80 Sugar Wheel Works
3808 N Williams Avenue, Suite 134, PORTLAND
Tel: 503-236-8511
www.sugarwheelworks.com
Custom wheel maker

B81 BIKEmpowered (Bike Empowered)
5035 NE 23rd Avenue, PORTLAND
Tel: 503-975-2391
www.bikempowered.com
Repair classes and bicycling events

B82 Swanson Thomas & Coon Attorneys
820 SW 2nd Avenue, Suite 202, PORTLAND
Tel: 503-228-5222
www.stc-law.com
Personal injury attorneys specializing in bicycles and pedestrians

B83 Everybody's Bike Rentals
NE Going Street and NE 19th Avenue, PORTLAND
Tel: 503-893-4513
www.pdxbikerentals.com
Bike Rentals in northeast Portland

B84 Portland Bike Station
515 SW 3rd Avenue, PORTLAND
Tel: 503-265-8068
www.portlandbikestation.org
Bike Rentals, repairs and storage

B85 Kerr Bikes/Wheel Fun Rentals
1020 SW Naito Parkway, PORTLAND
Tel: 503-808-9955
www.kerrbikes.org
Bike Rentals downtown Portland

B86 Pedal Bike Tour Rentals
133 SW 2nd Avenue, PORTLAND
Tel: 503-243-2453
www.pedalbiketours.com
Bike Rentals and tours by bike

Bike Shops & Rentals

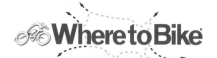 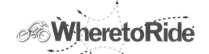

Also in this Series!

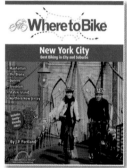

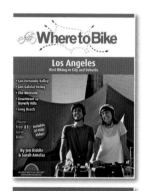

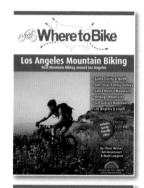

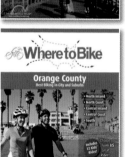

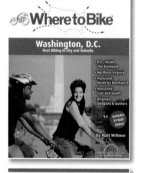

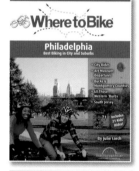

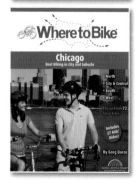

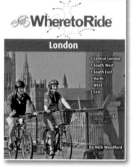

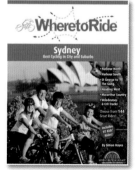

www.**WheretoBikeGuides**.com

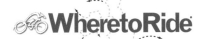 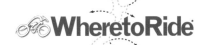

Also in this Series!

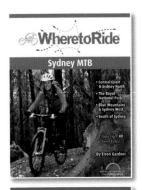

Sydney MTB
- Central Coast & Sydney North
- The Royal National Park
- Blue Mountains & Sydney West
- South of Sydney

Choose from 40 Great Rides!

By Erron Gardner

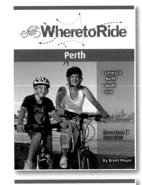

Perth
- Central & North
- South
- East

Choose from 43 great rides!

By Brent Meyer

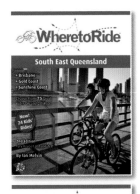

South East Queensland
- Brisbane
- Gold Coast
- Sunshine Coast

Choose from 75 Great Rides in this area!

New! 24 Kids' Rides!

2nd Edition

By Ian Melvin

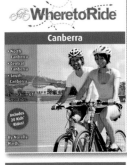

Canberra
- North Canberra
- Central Canberra
- South Canberra

Includes 20 Kids' Rides!

By Narelle Hards

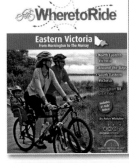

Eastern Victoria
From Mornington to The Murray
- North Eastern Victoria
- Around the Bays
- South Eastern Victoria

Choose from 88 Great Rides!

By Peter Whiteley

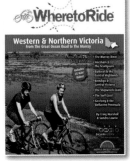

Western & Northern Victoria
From The Great Ocean Road to The Murray
- The Murray River
- Horsham & The Grampians
- Ballarat & the Central Highlands
- Bendigo & Central Victoria
- The Shipwreck Coast
- The Surf Coast
- Geelong & the Bellarine Peninsula

By Craig Marshall & Sandra Lowrie

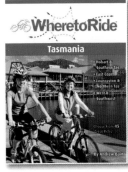

Tasmania
- Hobart & Southern Tas
- East Coast
- Launceston & Northern Tas
- West & Southwest

Choose from 45 Great Rides!

By Andrew Bain

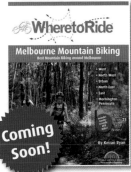

Melbourne Mountain Biking
Best Mountain Biking around Melbourne
- West
- North West
- Urban
- North East
- East
- Mornington Peninsula

Choose from 71 Rides!

By Keiran Ryan

Coming Soon!

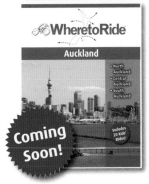

Auckland
- North Auckland
- Central Auckland
- South Auckland

Includes 20 Kids' Rides!

Coming Soon!

www.**WheretoBikeGuides**.com

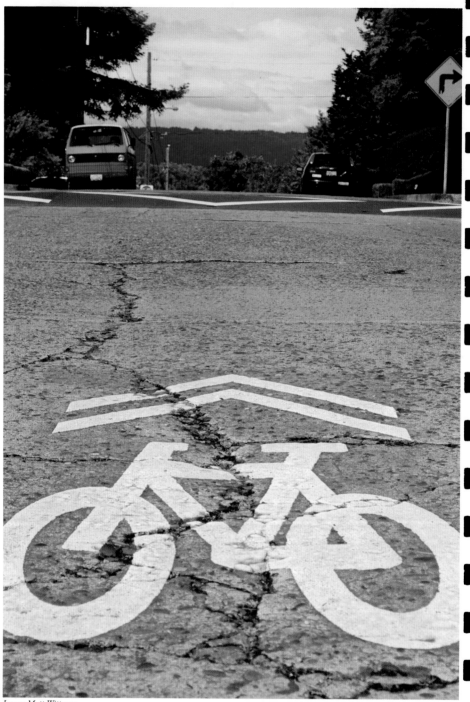

Image Matt Wittmer